W9-CNL-734

BACK PAIN

What Works!

A Comprehensive Guide
to Preventing and Overcoming
Back Problems

Joseph Kandel, M.D.
David B. Sudderth, M.D.

PRIMA PUBLISHING

© 1996 by Joseph Kandel and David B. Sudderth

All rights reserved. No part of this book may be reproduced or transmitted in any form or by any means, electronic or mechanical, including photo-copying, recording, or by any information storage or retrieval system, without written permission from Prima Publishing, except for the inclusion of quotations in a review.

PRIMA PUBLISHING and its colophon are trademarks of Prima Communications, Inc.

Library of Congress Cataloging-in-Publication
Kandel, Joseph.
    Back pain—what works! / by Joseph Kandel and David Sudderth.
       p.   cm.
    Includes bibliographical references and index.
    ISBN 0-7615-0327-7
    1. Backache—Popular works.   I. Sudderth, David B.   II. Title.
RD771.B217K36   1996
    617.5'64—dc20   95-54092
                                                            CIP

99 DD 10 9 8 7 6 5 4 3 2
Printed in the United States of America

All products mentioned in this book are trademarks of their respective companies.

The illustrations in chapters 1, 2, and 4, with the exception of Figures 2-2, 2-8, and 2-9, are reprinted with permission of The Sign Shop and the Med X Corporation.

Warning—Disclaimer
The information provided in this book is not intended to be a substitute for professional or medical advice. The author and publisher specifically disclaim any liability, loss or risk, personal or otherwise, which is in-curred as a result, directly or indirectly, of the use and application of any of the contents of this book.

How to Order
Single copies may be ordered from Prima Publishing, P.O. Box 1260, Rocklin, CA 95677; telephone (916) 632-4400. Quantity discounts are also available. On your letterhead, include information concerning the in-tended use of the books and the number of books you wish to purchase.

Visit us online at http://www.primahealth.com

To my wife, Merrylee, thank you for everything that you do. I love you.

—Joseph Kandel

To my partner, my patients, and my dear friend Alan Mengel, whose thoughtfulness and encouragement have provided focus and clarity to this project.

—David B. Sudderth

Contents

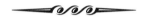

Acknowledgment

W̲e would like to thank Chris Adamec for her assistance in the research and proofreading of our manuscript.

Introduction

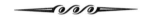

You can't concentrate, you can't do your job well, and you've even cut back (or given up) on sex. That pain in your back can put you out to pasture, whether you're thirty or sixty. But it doesn't have to be that way! We're physicians who are experts on back pain, and we want to tell you that the worst thing you can do is accept back pain as your lot in life. In most cases, there's plenty that you and your doctor can do to resolve—or at least improve—the problem.

Back pain is one of the most pervasive medical problems in our society, and it's also an equal opportunity kind of pain, affecting both men and women, as well as people of all socioeconomic strata, ages, races, and ethnic groups. About 80 percent of Americans will experience at least one incident of severe back pain in their lives. And for about 20 percent of them, that pain will become chronic, interfering with work, family life, and even sexual pleasure.

This book provides important advice on how to alleviate the back pain that you and your loved ones suffer. Even if your back has bothered you for years, you will discover that it's possible to live a more comfortable, active life.

While individuals obviously must cope with the financial and psychological costs of back pain in their daily lives, society also pays a high price for the problem. According to the January 1994 issue of *The Back Letter,* the direct medical costs of back pain are about $25 billion. Add to that another $25 billion to $75 billion in indirect costs—disability costs, lost work time, and diminished productivity—and you're looking at an extremely expensive problem.

Furthermore, back pain imposes a great deal of downtime on many sufferers. Americans spend nearly three million days in hospital beds each year because of back pain problems, and studies indicate that most of these people are not elderly. The first baby boomers turned fifty in 1996, and as this large segment of the population ages, the incidence of back pain will increase.

Another aspect of the back pain problem is our increasingly sedentary lives. Remote-control television, drive-through banks, and many more time-saving devices are actually contributing to the problem. We are far less active than our parents were at our age, and *they* are less active than their parents were at the same age. And a sedentary lifestyle contributes directly to back pain.

Here's how it works: Your back hurts, so you rest, often for many more days than you need to. You decondition your back, and it hurts more. So you rest more. Soon you're in a downward spiral of pain and frustration. The solution is to develop an understanding of what's going on with your body and to follow a simple exercise program that works, combined with proper medical advice.

A Real Problem

Too many patients and their doctors consider back pain as worthy of no more than cursory treatment and, instead, believe it should be accepted as an unpleasant fact of life. Some physicians will actually tell patients that the problem is an inevitable result of humans walking upright—we've evolved too highly from the knuckle-dragger stage.

Even if that were true—and we would argue that it's irrelevant because people do walk upright and have for many thousands of years—does it mean we must accept back pain as our lot in life? Is it a basic condition of being human?

Our answer to these questions is an unqualified no. We ardently disagree with those who feel that back pain is unimportant or can't be decreased. Nor do we believe back pain should be passively accepted. As neurologists, we aggressively treat back pain with as much enthusiasm as other specialists treat cancer or heart disease.

Why? Because we know that if back pain is ignored, it can lead to serious medical problems, including deterioration of the lungs and heart, obesity from inaction (which leads to additional physical problems), arthritis, and many other illnesses. Moreover, patients with acute or chronic back pain feel miserable and out of control. They can't handle their usual activities at work, they can't play with their kids at home, and even their sex lives may be impaired. *Don't let this happen to you!*

We want to put the patient back in control. In this book, we advise you on how to identify a caring and knowledgeable physician, and we explain the treatments that are available today to diminish or eliminate your back pain. We also discuss the latest diagnostic methods for back problems. We talk about the importance of exercise and provide simple and yet extremely effective exercises that you will note rapid improvement from doing. We know every excuse in the book for not exercising—and we can counter them all!

Motivation is important, too, and we'll talk about why you should regain control of your life and how you can do so. Too many people have suffered for too many years when help was available.

How to Use This Book

We recommend that you read every chapter, although we understand that some readers will immediately turn to information about medications or the anatomy of the back, while others will be more interested in non-pharmacological treatments and still others may be intrigued by the chapter on sexual satisfaction and a bad back.

Whatever your particular interests, be sure to read chapter 5, which describes specific exercises to improve your back. And if you or a loved one needs surgery, you'll find valuable information in chapter 8, which covers the latest high-tech options as well as more traditional treatments. We also discuss your back and your sex life (chapter 9), sports and your back (chapter 10), and how to travel with minimum discomfort to your back (chapter 11).

The section titled "Frequently Asked Questions," which begins on page 179, will interest most readers, because this is where we explore the questions that confuse and distress so many people.

Along with following the guidelines of this book, you must be under the care of a good doctor who knows your individual needs and health history. This physician should be caring and competent. If you need to find a new doctor, chapter 3 explains what kinds of doctors treat people with low back pain and how you can find the best physician for your problem.

As we wrote this book, we tried not to use cumbersome medical terminology, but sometimes it couldn't be avoided. For this reason, we've provided a glossary (which begins on page 189) to clarify any terms that may be unfamiliar to you and not fully explained within the chapters themselves.

Conclusion

We can't promise to rid you of low back pain forever, but we can offer you numerous suggestions on how to reduce its duration and severity. Don't accept the pain! Fight back! Use our book as a tool in your arsenal of weapons against this disease. Our advice can help you regain control and enjoyment of your own life. You don't have to suffer anymore.

1

Causes of Back Pain

———◦/◦/◦———

Your back hurts for a reason (or maybe for several reasons). This reason, or cause, is the first thing your doctor seeks to discover. After making a diagnosis, he or she can treat the problem and, hopefully, return you to a pain-free existence. This chapter covers various causes of back pain, from the most common to the relatively rare.

The Most Common Cause of Back Pain

As outlined by Dr. A. Melleby in *The Y's Way to a Healthy Back*, a great deal of evidence suggests that for more than 80 percent of individuals with subacute or chronic low back pain, the cause is weak trunk muscles. Rarely is there a severe underlying structural abnormality, although the two are not necessarily separate. A number of conditions—a degenerated or inflamed joint, degenerative disease of the spine, degenerative disease of a disc, or inflammation of various components of the spinal column—can cause impaired mobility of the spine muscles and lead to a weakened state. Experts in industrial medicine have long known that weak low back muscles are a significant risk factor for low back problems.

A study published in the respected medical journal *Spine,* by Dr. Panjabi and others, found that a cadaver's spine, when the muscles had been removed, could carry only five pounds or less before it began to buckle. This clearly shows that the muscles provide most of the spinal column's strength. (See the next chapter to learn about the anatomy of the spine.)

Thus it is important that we look at the roles that the lumbar (low back) support muscles play. Weak muscles contribute to chronic back pain and a deconditioned state. Strong muscles aid in resisting injury and preventing abnormal motion, which causes pain.

The Many Possible Causes of Back Pain

In the next chapter, we'll look at the basic structure of the back, and you'll see how relatively simple the lower spine actually is. Our model will allow you to comprehend the multitude of causes of both acute and chronic low back pain.

To determine the best treatment for an individual patient, a physician must consider the wide variety of potential causes of back pain in that patient. It helps a lot when you, as an informed patient, understand the anatomy of your spine; you can then logically consider your symptoms and also draw useful conclusions about the possible causes of your pain.

Unfortunately, unlike many other types of illness, low back pain does not work very well on a conventional medical model. Such models are based on the assumption that there is a precisely identifiable structural problem and if a doctor can find this problem, then he or she can treat it, and the illness will be resolved. For example, the medical model would indicate that the patient with pneumonia be given antibiotics— germs killed, problem solved.

Often there are multiple factors involved in low back pain, as has recently been discovered by most specialists dealing with spine pain disorders. Even with the most advanced technology, a clinician may fail to discover the precise nature and source of the pain.

However, many people who suffer from low back pain try to pinpoint one or two causes for their problem, and they typically settle on the most frightening possibilities. Patients who come to our office with acute or chronic low back pain usually believe that their pain comes from either cancer or a ruptured disc. The good news is that while these two ailments can cause low back pain, they are by no means the most common causes.

We can separate the causes of back pain into the following categories: local anatomic conditions or diseases, diseases in the abdominal cavity, chemical changes, underlying ailments, infections, inflammatory conditions, and, of course, injuries.

All of these problems are known to lead to low back pain, with one additional category to be added: psychological factors. A growing number of researchers and doctors believe that stress and anxiety can aggravate and prolong back pain, even if they are not the underlying cause.

Local Anatomic Conditions or Diseases

This category of problems that can cause back pain includes the classic ruptured disc as well as arthritis, spinal stenosis, osteoporosis from loss of calcium, inflammation of the sacroiliac joint, fibromyalgia, and cancer.

Ruptured disc   Do you realize that in some ways the discs in your back are like jelly doughnuts? (Although, happily, they're much tougher.) This analogy may help you to understand that infamous disorder, a ruptured disc—or, in medical terms, a herniated nucleus pulposus. When your doctor says you have a ruptured disc, this means that the disc has torn open and released some of its gelatinous core (very much like the jelly inside the doughnut). The release can damage nerves or the structural integrity of the spine.

This problem rarely requires surgery. But if it's associated with progressive weakness or intractable pain, surgery may be an option you'll need to consider. (See chapter 8 for more information on this subject.)

What causes a disc to rupture? Many conditions can lead to this disorder, but it is clear that if the supporting structures of the spine are not kept strong, flexible, and intact, then the lower spine can become weak and unfit—more susceptible to injury. Along with this deterioration comes an instability of the structures that hold the joints of the spine in place, and this can result in the discs protruding or even rupturing (see Figure 1-1).

Of course, direct trauma (injury caused by something outside of the body), especially when the spine is stretched backward or forward or twisted to one side, can make a disc rupture or protrude as well. A car accident could conceivably lead to such a problem.

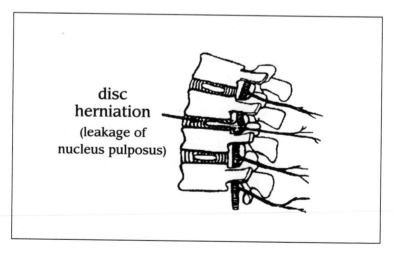

disc herniation
(leakage of nucleus pulposus)

Figure 1-1

Local Arthritis   Another possible cause of back pain is local arthritis, often the type associated with wear and tear on the joints. This is called osteoarthritis, or spondylosis when the spine is involved. When we are young, the segments of the spinal column are quite smooth and regular, but as we age, bone spurs (abnormal bony projections) and other changes occur, and they may actually create jagged edges on the vertebrae. These edges can cause pain and irritation in your low back. In addition, the jagged edges can cause a misalignment of your vertebrae, and if a vertebra is off center, you may feel pain.

Spinal Stenosis   A degenerative disorder that is frequently misdiagnosed or missed altogether, spinal stenosis occurs when the central canal of the spine (where the nerves lie) becomes narrowed, possibly due to the natural degeneration of the bones with age or to bone spurs that accompany degenerative changes. When this state occurs, there is less room for the nerve roots to exit through the openings between the vertebrae, and the pressure can cause the nerve roots to become acutely inflamed. People with spinal stenosis may experience a sensation of numbness and burning in both legs. (This has often been misdiagnosed as neuropathy, which is an irritation of the small nerve fibers in the legs.) Sometimes spinal stenosis occurs after a person has had back surgery. Most of the people who have spinal stenosis are over the age of fifty.

Osteoporosis   Another cause of back pain may be a loss of calcium in the bones, which can soften and change the shape of the spine. This is called osteoporosis of the spine. The softening may also lead to unnatural fractures of the spinal column, and this, too, can cause pain.

The Sacroiliac Joint   What exactly is the sacroiliac joint? Basically, it is the joint between the tailbone and the pelvic girdle. This is a site that experiences a great deal of wear and tear, causing changes to the lower spine as well as to the pelvis.

In the past, almost every type of acute or chronic pain that was associated with the low back was called "sacroiliac pain," referring to the sacroiliac joint. This diagnostic term has fallen out of favor over the last few years, and doctors seldom use it.

However, the diagnosis does have validity, as documented in an article by Dr. A. Schwarzer that appeared in a 1995 issue of *Spine*. In an extensive evaluation of patients with chronic low back pain, Schwarzer found that he could significantly reduce their complaints of discomfort by using local injections to numb the affected area and reduce inflammation at the joint. This excellent study highlights the fact that chronic low back pain is a direct result of inflammation of the sacroiliac joint in anywhere from 9 to 30 percent of patients with this type of pain. The study also proves that past ways of thinking about a problem aren't always wrong, and their validity may be worth considering. In other words, "Everything old is new again."

Pain from the sacroiliac joint often worsens with sitting as well as with walking or standing, so doctors have a hard time distinguishing it from other anatomic causes of low back pain. In our practice, we see inflammation of the sacroiliac joint more often as a cause of chronic low back pain, rather than acute pain. So if you suffer from chronic low back pain, the sacroiliac joint should be investigated as a possible source.

Fibromyalgia   Supporting structures of the low back region, such as muscles, tendons, and ligaments, can contribute to back pain. In particular, the very small muscles at the base of the spine, the spinal erector muscles, have to work constantly to keep us upright. These muscles can become acutely inflamed, which can lead to irritation and inflammation of the coverings of the muscles.

This muscle covering is called the myofascial sheath, and it's very much like the sheath that you have probably seen on a chicken breast that you bought at the supermarket and prepared at home. You cannot cut or chew through the chicken muscle sheath; the sheaths of our own muscles are similarly tough.

One problem is that these sheaths have a very poor blood supply, and if they become inflamed, they can stay inflamed and painful for a long period of time. Doctors may refer to this condition as myofascial pain, fibromyalgia, or fibromyositis. It is quite difficult to treat.

Cancer   Medically known as neoplasm, cancer is a structural disease that may cause back pain. While cancer in the back would most commonly result from a metastatic change (originating somewhere else and spreading to the spine), there are also rare episodes of cancer that begin within the spinal cord or around the nerve root. Rarely, cancer can begin in the bony spinal column itself.

Abdominal Cavity Diseases

A variety of internal illnesses can lead to or cause low back pain. These include kidney disease and ulcers or pancreatic problems. One extremely serious illness is an aneurysm in the abdominal aorta—the large artery that supplies the abdomen and legs with oxygen-rich blood.

Aneurysm   When the aorta is enlarged with a bubblelike formation that pouches out, it should be considered a medical emergency. Very much like a bubble on the inner tube of a tire, a bleb that occurs on the large artery is called an aneurysm and can cause severe stabbing or shooting pains in the low back. Pain may also radiate down both legs. This can affect the blood flow not only to the legs but also to the kidneys, and as a result the person may feel pain in the sides between the ribs and hips. Never ignore such sensations.

In addition, there are a number of organs in the abdominal cavity, and any one of them can develop cancer. This is not the most likely cause of back pain, but it needs to be a consideration because of the gravity of such an illness.

Kidney Disorders   Kidney disease, as well as inflammation of the ureters (the tubes that go from the kidney to the bladder), can cause pain in the low back area. Often people with kidney or bladder infections experience severe low back pain. This is called referred pain.

Referred pain is pain felt in a place other than its source. You probably know that someone suffering a heart attack will experience pain, numbness, or heaviness in the left arm, along with crushing chest pain. This is obviously not a problem with the person's left arm. In a similar fashion, pain can be referred from the abdominal cavity to the low back and down to the legs.

Ulcers and Pancreatic Problems   A stomach or duodenal ulcer may cause pain and a burning, knifelike sensation in the lower spine. This kind of pain may also be experienced if the pancreas becomes inflamed. The pancreas is a small organ that produces insulin, which controls sugar levels in the bloodstream. When a tumor, scarring, alcohol abuse, or another problem causes inflammation in a person's pancreas, he or she may feel pain in the low back area. This is another example of referred pain.

It's interesting, however, that colon inflammation rarely causes referred pain in the low back area. As a rule, symptoms of colon inflammation are abdominal cramping, stomach irritation, and changes in bowel habits.

Chemical Causes

Chemical changes in the body may manifest themselves as many different illnesses. In the spine, a change such as an increase in the level of uric acid, which is associated with gout, can produce spine inflammation and severe arthritis-like pain in the joints.

As previously mentioned, changes in insulin or glucose (sugar) in the bloodstream can cause all sorts of changes in the nervous system. One of the more common of these is inflammation of the little nerve fibers, usually in the arms and legs. This is called neuropathy, meaning a distortion of information sent from the nerve to the body and brain. Neuropathy can produce virtually any type of sensory disturbance, but it often causes pain in the legs and can cause pain in the lower spine as well. It's a sharp, stabbing, burning, aching, squeezing, gripping, or tearing sensation.

In addition, there is a relatively uncommon disorder of the spine called Paget's disease, in which the bones will weaken and then break, reheal, break again, and reheal again. During this process, small nerve fibers can be trapped inside healing bones, which can be extremely painful. An individual with this condition may feel pain in the spine, buttocks, or legs.

Underlying Ailments

Any time a person has an illness, his or her nervous system works less efficiently. Therefore, if someone has a spine disorder such as inflammation, arthritis, or joint changes, and then he or she develops a medical problem (perhaps heart, lung, kidney, or liver disease), the increased inflammation will likely cause more pain. This feeling will usually return to its normal state of chronic pain when the other medical problem has been resolved.

Infections

Although infection is not a common cause of back pain, it is a very important consideration when you and your doctor are trying to determine why your back hurts. People who have AIDS or any other chronic illness and people who have been taking steroids may have suppressed immune systems. For them, the symptoms of infection are not always fever, chills, and warmth over the infected area.

This is particularly true when a disc is infected (diskitis), since this condition produces few signs or symptoms of illness besides back pain. Likewise, if there is an infection in the bony spine called osteomyelitis, the person may feel vague, nondescript pain in the lower spine. Nevertheless, the infection needs to be diagnosed and treated with antibiotics if the pain is to come under control. Not only that, if left untreated, this infection can spread along the spinal column, leading to more serious problems.

A form of infection surrounding the spinal sac is called an epidural abscess. This is known in medical literature as the "great imitator" because, like tuberculosis and syphilis, it can produce a great variety of symptoms. The low back may ache, but low-grade, fluctuating fever; malaise; fatigue; and joint pains are other possible symptoms. When seeking to diagnose back pain, this possibility must be considered, particularly in a person who has a compromised immune system.

An epidural abscess is treated surgically. The doctor opens the low back spine, allowing the pus to drain, and then gives antibiotics to fight the infection.

An additional consideration is meningitis, which is often called "spinal meningitis." The most common form is a viral (nonbacterial) infection; if you drink plenty of fluids and rest in bed, it passes quickly. Bacterial meningitis is more serious. After a diagnosis is made, it needs to be treated aggressively with antibiotics, fluids, and vigilant medical supervision. If untreated, bacterial meningitis frequently results in death.

The symptoms of meningitis may appear gradually and worsen slowly, which can interfere with making a prompt diagnosis. If a person has stiffness in the neck, back, and legs, along with fever; if he or she looks ill; or if he or she has an elevated white blood cell count, spinal meningitis is a possibility. This illness must be treated correctly and quickly to avoid long-term complications, such as scarring of the nerve roots (which itself causes pain). This is discussed in the following section.

Inflammatory Conditions

Inflammation is the body's response to a wide variety of problems. True inflammatory arthritic conditions (in contrast to osteoarthritis, which is probably a wear-and-tear process)— for example, rheumatoid arthritis—can affect not only the fingers, the wrists, the elbows, and the large joints, but also the joints of the lower spine. Protracted inflammation from many different disorders can often be treated with anti-inflammatory medicines, heat, exercise, and muscle relaxant therapy. More potent drugs are occasionally required, however.

While inflammatory disorders sometimes mimic acute infectious disorders, there is a significant difference in medical treatment for the two types. Therefore careful diagnosis is essential.

As previously mentioned, an inflammatory or, more likely, an infectious event may cause the nerve roots in the spinal column to become inflamed and clump together. This condition is known as arachnoiditis. Surgery that causes scars to form may also lead to this problem. In arachnoiditis, the nerve roots adhere to each other and become irritated, sending messages of pain up to the brain and down to the legs.

This is similar to the problem with adhesions women may experience following abdominal surgery or surgery on the reproductive organs. (An adhesion is an abnormal, scar-related attachment of adjacent organs.) Women experiencing pain due to adhesions may need a second or even a third operation to sever the adhesions so they won't lead to a bowel obstruction or another painful problem.

Unfortunately, unlike abdominal or pelvic surgery for adhesions, low back surgery to reduce scar formation often leads to additional scar formation, which then leads to a more painful state. The good news is that it may be possible to correct this problem in the future through laser surgery, which can disintegrate the scar tissue. However, the jury is still out, and this is not yet a widely accepted or available treatment for arachnoiditis. (See the section on new surgical techniques in chapter 8 for more information on surgery that can limit scarring.)

Injuries

This is one of the largest categories of back pain causes. Whether the trauma has an obvious cause (such as falling down the stairs, having a car accident, or lifting a heavy piece of equipment), or whether it's a subtle deconditioned state that has affected the low back spine over a series of months or years (usually from decreased activity), the fact is that trauma accounts for numerous cases of low back pain.

Far and away the most common type of trauma is the simple muscle or ligament sprain. On a microscopic level, this injury involves the tearing of the smallest muscle or other tissue fibers, which leads to microscopic bleeding, which in turn produces swelling and local pain.

Although people commonly talk about having strains and sprains, in truth, a physician cannot be certain that this condition has occurred without doing a muscle biopsy (which is almost never done). Yet a fine clinician can diagnose a sprain by evaluating the change in muscle tone, the swelling or fluid content of the muscle, and how spongy or "boggy" the muscle seems. In addition, a patient often has associated injuries, such as muscle spasm in the initially unaffected muscles. These undamaged muscles are attempting to compensate for an injured muscle that is not doing its share of the work.

If, for example, a person hurts one hip and consequently walks with a different, pain-reducing gait over a period of weeks, pretty soon the other hip, the low back region, and the whole pelvic girdle become sore. In a similar fashion, when one muscle becomes inflamed, other muscles will often go into spasm, contracting tightly to compensate and protect the hurt muscle, thereby building up waste products and toxins that cannot be washed away because of high pressure in the tissues. The protecting muscle is thus secondarily inflamed. An unfortunate cycle is set in motion as both muscles try to protect each other, becoming more inflamed and painful.

Another injury that causes back pain is an acute fracture of the spine, which can lead to an unstable spine or even rotation of the spine. If the lower spine rotates, or bends too far forward or backward, the exiting nerve roots may be crushed, severed, or even irreversibly injured. (The discussion of anatomy in chapter 2 will help to clarify this.)

Moreover, the fracture alone—even without abnormal, nerve-damaging movement of the spine—causes pain that ranges in severity from dull and annoying all the way to severe and unbearable. As you know, different people have different levels of pain perception and different pain thresholds; therefore two individuals may have entirely different responses to similar injuries.

Psychological Factors

As we noted at the beginning of the chapter, psychological factors do play a role in back conditions. Back pain usually diminishes a person's enjoyment of daily activities, which has definite psychological consequences. Anyone who has ever had persistent back pain or lived with an individual who suffers from chronic back pain knows how difficult it is to accomplish things and to feel positive on a daily basis when your back hurts. A person's back pain often precludes enjoyable activities, including social events, which is also frustrating for the sufferer's partner. Just as illnesses such as ulcers typically have both physical and psychological components, so does back pain.

With the increase in stress that accompanies back pain, there is frequently also an increased muscle dysfunction. That can be spasm (increased muscle tightening), a limited range of motion of the lower spine, or even, over time, a loss of flexibility and function in the lower spine.

These related problems interact with the person's general emotional state, and, of course, when an individual has more pain, there is more stress and more anxiety. This may lead him or her into a downward spiral of negative emotions and negative physical responses. The more pain you have, the more anxious you become about having additional pain. And the more anxious you become, the more your muscles will tighten and the more restricted your range of motion will become.

Now you can see that if your back pain makes you depressed or irritable, and you subsequently feel even more pain, it's not "all in your head." There are real, physiological reasons for it. But don't despair. You can break out of this downward spiral. Medications and various therapies may help. Exercise can often improve your condition, too. In chapter 5, we discuss how to treat the classic deconditioned low back spine and end the cycle of anxiety and pain.

2

Understanding the Basic Anatomy of Your Back: A Working Model

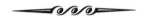

If you wish to combat your low back problem intelligently and effectively, a basic understanding of the anatomy of your back is essential. This may seem daunting to someone with no medical training. Many books on spinal problems, even those geared toward the general public, display confusingly complex diagrams featuring vertebrae, intervertebral discs, ligaments, the spinal cord, and the whole network of body parts involved with the spine. As a result, the problem seems far too complicated, and the reader sees no hope in trying to figure it all out.

We believe that knowledge is power, but we also believe that such excruciatingly difficult depictions of the back's intricacies are of little help to the average person. Therefore we've created a simple model that will help you to quickly grasp the basic structure of your back. You don't have to go to medical school to understand your back. This model will give you a rudimentary understanding of its anatomy, to help you make the right decisions about how to end your pain. After all, the more information you have, the more likely you are to obtain the care and treatment you need. You'll be able to ask your doctor the right questions and understand his or her answers.

The Rod Analogy

Forget for a moment how the human spine is actually constructed, and imagine that it is a rigid steel rod extending from the base of the skull to the tip of the tailbone.

Almost immediately, you can see that such a structure would cause serious problems and make daily living as we know it—even for those who already suffer from back pain—impossible. With a rigid metal spine, you could not, for example, bend at the waist, nor could you flex your neck forward or bend it backward. There could be no movement in the low back (lumbar spine).

In addition, your metal rod spine would not allow you to rotate. You couldn't turn your neck to one side or the other, so you would see only straight ahead, like a horse wearing blinders. Your hips couldn't rotate, limiting numerous activities—walking, dancing, lovemaking.

But these wouldn't be your only problems. One alarming problem would be the effect of any impact along the spine. Pressure exerted on the head, for example, would be immediately transmitted to the spine, sending shock waves down its entire length, into the pelvis and then the legs. Even gentle walking would cause this problem, while jumping and running would be intolerable.

Making the Rod Work

Clearly the rigid metal spine is unacceptable for many reasons. If we wanted to make it feasible, we would first need to divide the steel rod into small sections that would allow the back and neck to turn and bend. Also, some type of material should separate the rigid segments, allowing smooth movement and preferably also creating some absorption of shocks transmitted from the feet or head. Small rubber cylinders installed between the rigid sections of the rod would do the trick.

But this spine model still has some problems. For example, nothing is holding the whole structure together. Perhaps we could apply long strips of duct tape down the length of the spine, front and back. This would support the spine and help to hold it together.

Here's yet another problem: Where are we going to put the spinal cord? Encasement and protection of the spinal cord—the nervous tissue that runs from the brain down the back—are some of the most important functions of the human spine.

Why is it so important? Because the spinal cord conveys all information from the brain to the arms and legs, and all sensations from the arms and legs must go through the spinal cord to the brain. The spinal cord also conveys messages to the bowel, the bladder, and other organs. It is the original information superhighway! And just as the brain needs the skull's protection, the spinal cord is also extremely vulnerable to any type of pressure or deformation and therefore must be encased in a rigid compartment.

To make room for the spinal cord, we could, of course, bore a hole through the length of our modified metal spine. However, a different type of anatomic refinement would allow greater weight-bearing capacity and create a basis for additional articulations (joints) between adjacent vertebrae: If we placed a horseshoe-shaped arch at the back of each rigid segment of the spine, stacking the arches up, we would make a canal for the spinal cord. Moreover, there would be space for the nerve roots to exit between adjacent arches.

A bony prominence (articular processes; see Figure 2-1) could be placed at the top and bottom of each arch, allowing for the formation of two more joints between each pair of adjacent vertebrae. These projecting bones would provide resistance to excessive rotation or excessive forward or backward movement of individual segments, limiting the possibility of injury.

Our spinal model is proceeding well. But we must consider yet another problem: What will move this model? What will make it flex, extend, rotate, and bend from side to side?

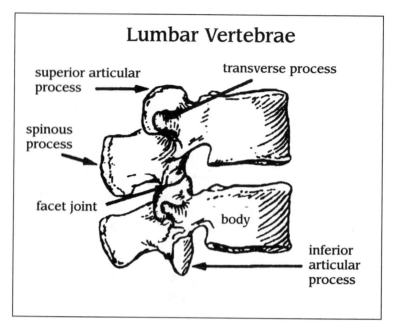

Lumbar Vertebrae

superior articular process

transverse process

spinous process

facet joint

body

inferior articular process

Figure 2-1

Of course, the only tissue that is able to move joints—and we can consider the spine to be a very complex joint—is muscle. Just as muscles move your knee or wrist, muscles move your spine. In order for the muscles to move the spine in so many ways, we have to place rigid structures on the arches to act as levers and attachment sites of the supporting musculature.

While this simplified construct has many anatomic short-comings, it analyzes the human spine quite correctly.

The Real Thing: Your Back

Having developed a model that brings us a better understanding of the basic anatomy and function of the human spine, let's move on to the real thing.

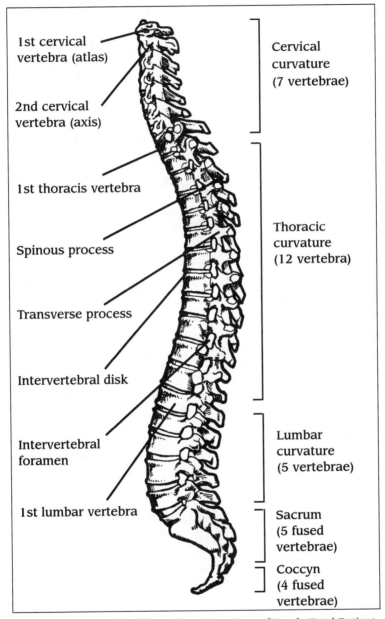

1st cervical
vertebra (atlas)

Cervical
curvature
(7 vertebrae)

2nd cervical
vertebra (axis)

1st thoracis vertebra

Spinous process

Thoracic
curvature
(12 vertebra)

Transverse process

Intervertebral disk

Intervertebral
foramen

Lumbar
curvature
(5 vertebrae)

1st lumbar vertebra

Sacrum
(5 fused
vertebrae)

Coccyn
(4 fused
vertebrae)

Figure 2-2 A model of the spine. *(Courtesy of Searle Total Patient Management Software V 1.0)*

A person's spine consists of similar, but not identical, bony elements stacked one on top of the other. (In our steel spine model, these were the small segments.) Each bony element is separated by an intervertebral disc (see Figure 2-3), which is made chiefly of cartilage. (Intervertebral discs were represented as small rubber cylinders in our model.)

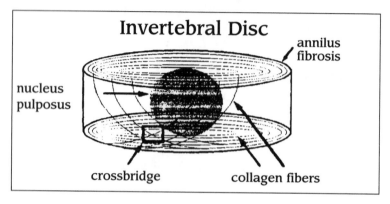

Invertebral Disc

annilus fibrosis

nucleus pulposus

crossbridge   collagen fibers

Figure 2-3

Doctors recognize five different sections of the spine. The cervical spine is the neck portion of the spine, comprising seven vertebrae. The thoracic, or rib-bearing portion of the spine, comprises twelve vertebrae. The lumbar spine (the low back) comprises five vertebrae. (See Figure 2-4.)

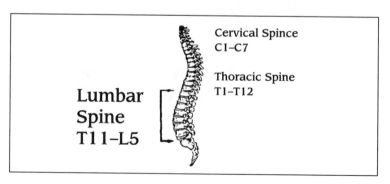

Cervical Spince
C1–C7

Thoracic Spine
T1–T12

Lumbar Spine T11–L5

Figure 2-4

Below the lumbar area is the sacrum, which connects to the pelvis and consists of five fused vertebrae. Attached to end of the sacrum is the coccyx, commonly called the tailbone. This lowest section of the spine is composed of four fused vertebrae.

The spine has curvatures that give it a springy quality, allowing it to bear loads more effectively by distributing the weight along its length. There are two types of curvatures: The lordosis is a gentle curving toward the front of the body, seen in the cervical spine and the lumbar spine. The kyphosis is a gentle curvature toward the back of the body, as in the thoracic spine.

Taking a look at the lumbar region, you'll see that the vertebrae here are somewhat larger than those in other portions of the spine and that the bony projection is at the back of the human body. The vertebral body is kidney shaped (see Figure 2-5), curving in slightly on both of its longer sides. The lumbar region is the main weight-bearing portion of the spine.

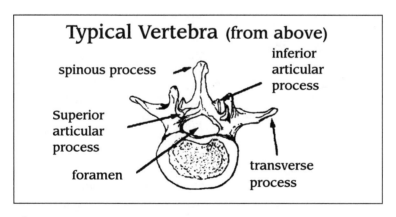

Typical Vertebra (from above)

spinous process

inferior articular process

Superior articular process

foramen

transverse process

Figure 2-5

A bony arch extends from one rounded portion of the vertebral body to the other, leaving an oval hole (foramen). These holes in the stacked vertebrae form the spinal canal. A pair of bony prominences extends outward from the arch, and another pair extends to the sides.

When you view the entire spine, you see that adjacent vertebrae form joints with one another. There are two separate joints, called facet joints, between two neighboring vertebrae. Facet joints are important structures because they are very potent pain generators in the human spine.

Take another look at Figure 2-5. A lever called a transverse process is on each side of a vertebra. (A *process* is simply a projecting part of a bodily structure.) One bony lever, the spinous process, extends backward. These levers are the individual knobs on your spine that you can feel through your skin, much like the bony projections visible on a dinosaur's spine. This can result in the pain that you may have felt directly under your skin at the midline of the spine when the bones, joints, ligaments, tendons, or muscles are inflamed. Levers are often attachment sites for the soft tissue structures that move the spine.

The portion of the bony arch between the transverse process and the spinous process is the lamina. (And when a lamina is removed, it's a laminectomy.)

The spinal cord begins at the base of the brain and travels down through the spinal canal, a cylindrical space formed by the stacking of the vertebrae. The spinal cord ends approximately at the lower end of the lumbar region's second segment.

Various nerves attached to the end of the spinal cord continue down to the sacrum and exit at various levels between adjacent vertebrae. (The fused vertebrae of the sacrum are not separated by intervertebral discs.)

The vertebrae of the sacrum are quite broad at the top and narrow as they descend to where the coccyx is attached. This has an appearance much like an arrowhead. The sacrum is connected to the ilium, a bone at each side of the pelvis, forming the sacroiliac joint (SI).

Up and down the entire spine, large supporting ligaments extend along the front and back of the vertebral bodies, forming the anterior and posterior longitudinal ligaments. (This is the duct tape we discussed earlier in our spine model.) These ligaments are very important for the support of the spine. (There are also ligaments that connect the various parts of the vertebral segments, but they don't pertain to our discussion.)

The spine also receives aid from large muscle groups that attach to the various levers of the spine, helping to stabilize it. These muscles, known as the paraspinal musculature, extend from the base of the skull to the sacrum. In the past, most doctors had no idea of the great importance of these muscles in maintaining a healthy spine. In fact, any successful rehabilitation of the low back really must address the strengthening of this musculature.

Back to the Jelly Doughnut

As we explained earlier, positioned between each adjacent pair of lumbar vertebral bodies is an intervertebral disc. We have often likened this amazing structure to a jelly doughnut. An intervertebral disc is composed primarily of cartilage. This somewhat elastic tissue forms the tough, resilient outer portion of the disc, which contains a gelatinous material at its center. (A similar type of material makes up your earlobe.) The inner jelly (nucleus pulposus) has a very high content of water. Intervertebral discs provide vertebrae with cushioned support and function essentially as universal joints.

When the Doughnut Crumbles

If the cartilaginous portion of the disc wears down, the inner portion breaks through and presses on various structures in the spinal canal or on the exiting nerve roots. As we mentioned in chapter 1, this is called a herniated nucleus pulposus or, more commonly, a slipped or ruptured disc.

A person's symptoms will depend on how and where a disc ruptures. If a disc in the cervical portion of the spine herniates, the spinal cord can be injured, leading to weakness in the arms and legs (quadriparesis). If a disc herniates to the side, it may put pressure on exiting nerve roots, causing a pinched nerve.

It's important to know that the blood supply to the discs is significantly reduced by the time a person is about twenty years old. The disc is living tissue and, like any other living tissue, needs to receive nutrients and eliminate waste products. A disc functions much like a sponge: When relaxed, the disc's tissue allows nutrients to enter it, and when compressed, the tissue expels waste products. When we exercise, we literally feed our discs by enhancing the fluid flow that brings them the nourishment and cleansing they need.

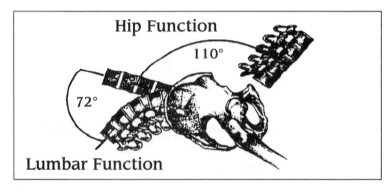

Figure 2-6 Hip rotation provides the first 110° of movement for the entire torso. Spine motion account for the remaining 72°.

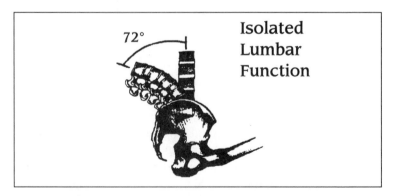

Figure 2-7 When the pelvis is stabilized and only spine motion is considered, there can be only a 72° range of motion.

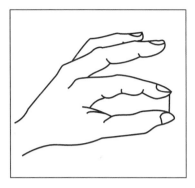

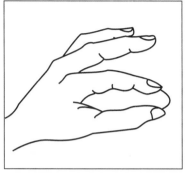

Figure 2-8 Your back is rigid when straight.

Figure 2-9 But once bent, it can help cushion the spine like a spring.

Another Analogy

Think of your back as a toothpick. In its normally straight state, it is strong and resistant to injury. It will transmit force delivered at one end efficiently, almost like a nail being driven into wood. A bent back has a spring-like quality and can cushion the levels of the spine. The curves of the normal spine reduce the degree of jarring that inevitably accompanies everyday life.

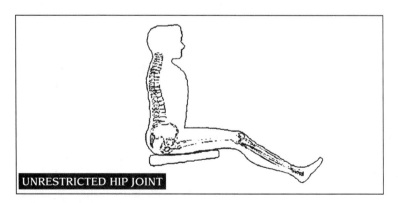

UNRESTRICTED HIP JOINT

Figure 2-10 A normal seated posture. Notice how the spine is positioned.

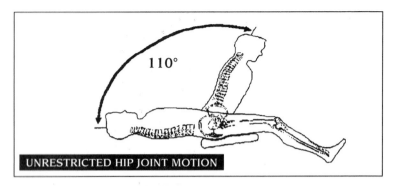

Figure 2-11 This shows the concept of motion due only to hip rotation. Notice how the spine retains the same alignment.

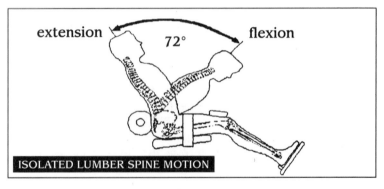

Figure 2-12 This illustrates the normal range of motion of the low back when the pelvis is stabilized.

Of course, the human spine is much more complex than either a steel rod or a wooden toothpick, and we have not considered all of the spine's elements in our discussion. But if you take the time to comprehend the simple model we have presented in this chapter, you will understand the terms and descriptions used by your doctor. You will not feel frustrated or excessively worried, and you can play an active role in making effective decisions about treatment. Empower yourself with information!

3

Types of Doctors and How to Choose a Good One

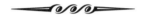

Where should you go to have your back pain treated? If you have an acute low back injury, a hospital's emergency room would be a reasonable starting place. This is not a good place to go, however, if your pain is chronic. In many facilities, you would be left waiting in an uncomfortable chair for hours and then get short shrift from the treating physician, whose goal is to get patients out of the emergency room as quickly as possible.

Of course, when your back has been aching for days or weeks, you may want to rush off to the first doctor who can see you, and, even without an appointment, an emergency room doctor might see you sooner than a busy specialist could. But it's far better to spend a little time gathering information, so you can find a physician who is right for you and your problem. In this chapter, we discuss medical doctors who treat people with chronic low back pain.

It's difficult to make generalizations about which branch of the medical profession deals most effectively with this ailment. A family practitioner in Racine, Wisconsin, might give a patient sounder advice than a neurosurgeon in Baltimore who did postgraduate training at Johns Hopkins. Our remarks on types of practitioners must be fairly general because doctors are individuals and hence there is great variation among them. Yet we can say with certainty that the ideal doctor is someone who is interested, compassionate, and well qualified.

When you're looking for a physician to treat your low back pain, try to keep an open mind, especially in the early phases of the search. If you think you'd prefer to see a certain type of doctor, such as a neurologist or an orthopedist, you'll probably find that many competent practitioners are available, but keep in mind that the doctor's specialty is not the only determining factor.

Your family practitioner is probably the best place to start your search for early treatment or a referral. But you should also talk to friends, relatives, neighbors, and acquaintances who have had chronic back problems. Ask them lots of questions about the physicians who treated them. If several people you know have good things to say about a particular doctor, you may want to make an appointment with him or her.

Be suspicious if the doctor you see cannot outline a plan for how your condition will be diagnosed or cannot set immediate and long-term treatment goals. If your low back pain is essentially the mechanical—that is, motion-related—type, without any symptoms involving your bowel, bladder, or legs, you should have serious doubts about a physician who orders an expensive test such as an MRI (magnetic resonance imaging) or an EMG (electromyography) on the first visit, or whose treatment plan doesn't go beyond recommending the use of an anti-inflammatory medication.

Do not remain with a physician whom you don't trust. The small amount of money invested in a second opinion is insignificant when you consider the long-term consequences of failed low back pain treatment. You need to have confidence in your doctor and believe that the proposed plan can help you. There are many qualified practitioners available. You simply have to search intelligently. The following list of questions may help you to determine whether a particular doctor is a good candidate for treating your back problem. Ask him or her:

1. About what percentage of your patients have low back pain? (If the doctor says it is 5 percent or less, you may wish to seek someone with more experience.)
2. Do you think that a person with low back pain can gain a lot of relief? (If the doctor says no and offers little hope, you may wish to seek another practitioner.)
3. Do you use medication to treat low back pain? (Most doctors use a variety of medications. It's a bad sign if the doctor refuses to use *any* medication.)
4. Do you think there is anything that a patient can do on his or her own to improve low back pain? If so, what are the options? (A doctor might recommend heat or exercise or a wide variety of choices. He or she should certainly have some ideas on what you can do to help yourself.)
5. If I have a flare-up of back pain, can I call you or your service, or do I have to go to the hospital emergency room? (It's a bad sign if the doctor says you must go to the ER when the clinic is closed.)

If you are in a managed care or HMO system, you may be referred to specific physicians. Generally, these doctors have been carefully screened. If you are unhappy with a doctor in the system, however, you often have the option to go "out of network" and pay a higher rate. Ask your insurance company for information about this.

Doctors Who Treat Without Surgery

Many nonsurgical branches of medicine deal with low back pain. As we said earlier in the chapter, the type of specialist is less important than the particular physician's interest in and approach to treating low back pain.

While we are aware that many surgeons try to manage their patients conservatively—that is, without performing surgery—in the beginning, we recommend starting your search with a doctor who does not do surgery. When you're in pain, it's easy to be convinced by an enthusiastic surgeon that you need an operation.

Family Practitioners

After medical school, family practitioners complete a residency training program of four years, during which time they are exposed to the diagnosis and treatment of essentially all types of medical and surgical conditions. They will treat your colds and your high blood pressure and may even deliver your baby. They also see a lot of back pain, as they are often the first stop in the process of getting treatment for acute and chronic low back problems. Many of them are very good at treating the more simple problems, and some of them may have developed effective regimens for treating people who suffer from low back pain. However, it is extremely difficult to remain current in all fields of medicine, and clearly many family practitioners are not informed with regard to the most up-to-date diagnostic and therapeutic options. If you are required to see a family practitioner by your HMO, or if you have an excellent family doctor whom you trust, this is a fine place to start.

Neurologists

These doctors diagnose and treat diseases of the nervous system. Because we are neurologists, we are familiar with the orientations and practicing styles of other members of our medical specialty. Consequently, we realize that many neurologists have little or no interest in treating patients with low back pain and are mainly interested in other nervous system problems. However, in terms of training, no other type of specialist is more qualified to treat problems of the lumbar spine.

Neurologists are extensively trained in pain theory, the bony anatomy of the spine, and the anatomy of the central and peripheral nervous systems. As a general rule, they also have considerable training in psychiatry and are well equipped to deal with the difficult emotional problems that accompany back pain. As you may know, these emotional problems can be as debilitating as the disorder itself.

After finishing medical school, the neurologist undergoes a four-year training period in the diseases of the nervous system. Typically, during this training, months are devoted to the study of neurosurgery, radiology, psychiatry, and rehabilitation. It's also important to note that neurologists are, in general, the practitioners who are most qualified to perform electromyography (a procedure that determines whether you have muscle or nerve root inflammation). Occasionally physiatrists (see next section) perform this study, but this study belongs primarily to the realm of neurology.

Many neurologists are highly skilled at interpreting the results of magnetic resonance imaging (MRI), a scanning procedure that shows the body's soft tissue structures and can reveal the location and type of injury. In fact, the MRI is the cornerstone of modern low back pain diagnosis. In addition, neurologists often perform many of the injections discussed later in this book. Usually, the directors of multidisciplinary pain centers are neurologists.

Physiatrists

Physiatrists treat disease and injury through physical means such as heat, electricity, and exercise. They tend to rely less on medications than other specialists. Physiatrists are medical doctors who have typically completed four years of postgraduate training in rehabilitative medicine. During this program, they study the treatment of conditions that require intensive rehabilitation, such as stroke and spinal cord injuries.

A physiatrist can be an excellent choice when you're looking for a doctor to treat your low back pain, but make sure he or she has access to the proper rehabilitative equipment, such as MedX or other strengthening equipment. Don't assume that your physiatrist has the best appliances or instruments for treating your problem. Ask questions to see whether he or she stays up to date on the latest equipment and methods.

Rheumatologists

After finishing medical school, a rheumatologist completes a three-year fellowship in internal medicine. During this very demanding program, the doctor is trained in essentially all fields of internal medicine, including cardiology, pulmonology, and gastroenterology (study of the heart, the lungs, and the digestive system, respectively). After this, the physician does a two-year fellowship in which he or she studies joint diseases.

A rheumatologist treats such disorders as rheumatoid arthritis, lupus, osteoarthritis, and many other conditions involving joint inflammation. This type of practitioner tends to rely quite heavily on the use of anti-inflammatory medications (which we discuss in chapter 6). These medications might by taken orally or given by injection into the joints.

Other Possible Sources of Help

Anesthesiologists   These physicians are frequently involved in the treatment of low back problems because their work directly addresses pain. Another doctor may refer you to an anesthesiologist for specific procedures, such as nerve blocks, facet blocks, and epidural steroid injections.

Spine Centers   When you're suffering from low back pain, the idea of going to a "spine center" sounds perfectly reasonable. We do not recommend this, however. While there are probably spine centers that provide efficient and quality care for low back pain, we have rarely had good experiences with these meccas. Often their greatest strengths are in their marketing strategies! Many of these institutions simply herd crowds of patients through a labyrinth of expensive studies and exposure to numerous medical specialists, none of whom has a guiding hand in any individual's treatment. At the end of the evaluation and therapy, the patient gets an operation or is declared cured—whether or not he or she agrees with that statement—or else the patient is told that he or she must learn to live with the pain. Although a spine center presents a theoretical advantage in that you would see a number of different specialists, we believe that you would be dissatisfied with the results.

Surgeons

Surgeons are in a class of their own. They have specialized in surgery because they believe in its curative powers and enjoy practicing it. As a general rule, if a surgeon doesn't feel that your condition calls for surgical intervention, he or she won't continue to treat you. The two types of surgeons who deal with low back pain are orthopedic surgeons and neurosurgeons, and we discuss them in the following subsections.

Many people seem to believe that unnecessary surgeries are commonly performed in the United States. But in our experience, this rarely happens on a conscious basis. Rather, in good faith, an overzealous surgeon performs an operation that another medical professional might reasonably argue is not required for the patient's ailment. Consequently, when it comes to consulting surgeons and considering invasive procedures, your personal involvement in your medical care is of great importance. You may also wish to obtain a second or even a third opinion on whether surgery would truly improve your condition. (In chapter 8, we discuss the circumstances under which surgery is a reasonable option.)

Orthopedists

An orthopedist, or orthopedic surgeon, is a medical doctor who has completed an orthopedic surgical residence, typically of four years. The orthopedist will commonly also have done a period of post-residency fellowship training in some specific aspect of orthopedic surgery. Orthopedists deal primarily with bone fractures, joint replacement, and similar problems. Competition for orthopedic surgery residencies is fierce. The individuals who go into this profession tend to be very intelligent and gifted with great manual dexterity.

If you go to an orthopedist, his or her evaluation will focus on determining whether your condition is one that surgery could potentially cure or relieve. Orthopedists frequently remove slipped discs and carry out a procedure called spinal fusion that allows two vertebrae to grow together where a diseased disc used to be. If the orthopedist does not diagnose such a condition, he or she will likely prescribe nonsteroidal anti-inflammatory medications and physical therapy.

Besides treating low back problems, the orthopedic surgeon generally does hip and other joint replacements as well as orthoscopic surgery (minor procedures done through a small incision with indirect visualization using a flexible "flashlight," or endoscope).

Neurosurgeons

Orthopedic surgeons and neurosurgeons do the same operations, so the issue is not which type of surgeon to see but which individual doctor to choose.

Neurosurgeons are medical doctors who have done postgraduate surgical training, during which they learned all the varieties of surgical procedures but spent most of their time in neurosurgery. These physicians not only surgically treat herniated discs and spinal stenosis, but they also operate on brain tumors and other disorders involving the nervous system. Like orthopedic surgeons, neurosurgeons seek to detect conditions that can be corrected through surgery.

Nonmedical Sources of Help

Many kinds of nonmedical practitioners treat back pain with non-pharmacologic methods. These practitioners include acupuncturists, massage therapists, and biofeedback experts (usually psychologists). In chapter 7, we discuss these treatment options in detail.

Chiropractors

Chiropractors are doing something right. They have hordes of satisfied patients who swear by chiropractic and reject the advice of most medical physicians to avoid the chiropractic profession. We think chiropractic is a good therapeutic option for many patients with back pain. Over the years, we have had experience with many chiropractors and receive numerous referrals from them. We also send patients to chiropractors on a regular basis.

Chiropractors go through a demanding and thorough training program. The graduates of chiropractic school leave with a grasp of the anatomy of the spine and nervous system as well as the various techniques relevant to spinal disorders. They are also taught when they should *not* adjust patients. Despite sharing many thousands of patients with chiropractors, we are unable to report a single injury received by one of our patients while being adjusted.

As chiropractors cannot give oral medications or injections, they frequently co-manage the more difficult patients with MDs. Chiropractic's safety and efficacy have become more widely acknowledged within the medical establishment in recent times.

Conclusion

Choosing a health care provider may seem like a daunting task, but if you spend a little time reviewing this chapter, talk to friends and relatives who have been treated for chronic back problems, and carefully consider your own concerns and desires about treatment, then you can make a choice that literally changes your life. We hope that this overview has helped you to understand the nature and orientation of the various medical specialists, as well as providing some guidance on what you should consider as you go about your search.

4

The Back Exam

W hat should you expect to happen when you go to see a doctor about chronic low back pain? In this chapter, we will tell you about the medical history that the doctor will take, about the examination itself, and about various tests that the doctor may order, depending on the results of your examination. It can be extremely helpful to know what to expect, both to be prepared and to alleviate any fears you have.

Assumptions and Fears

After having been in a car accident, a very pleasant thirty-two-year-old woman was referred to our office from the local hospital. An ambulance had taken her to the emergency room, where a doctor had examined her, x-rays had been taken, and a diagnosis of "back strain" was pronounced. She was then told she needed a neurologist's assessment and care.

This woman accepted the ambulance ride and the ER visit as normal consequences of having been in a car accident. But

41

when the ER doctor told her that she needed neurologic assessment, she became anxious. At the end of the evaluation with Dr. Kandel, she explained, "I thought there must be something very wrong, something [the ER doctor] was hiding from me, or else I wouldn't have to see a neurologist."

During the initial discussion, she repeatedly asked, "Do you want me to sit on the exam table?" despite Dr. Kandel's assurance that he preferred to have her sitting in a chair, where she could be more relaxed and hence more able to provide information on her symptoms and history. Next Dr. Kandel examined her, and he then explained what was probably wrong and what he thought she would experience in terms of her symptoms over the next days and weeks. Before she left, the patient said, "I was more scared about seeing a neurologist than I was about my back pain!"

This story illustrates that patients come to their appointments with very different expectations as well as many different concerns and anxieties. All these ideas and feelings work together to play a significant role in a patient's illness. Thus, if you can be relaxed and prepared for your doctor's visit, you'll find it easier both to explain your symptoms and problems and to answer the doctor's questions. You will be facilitating the diagnosis as well as your treatment. Fear and foreboding, on the other hand, can impair the whole process.

The Initial Discussion

Regardless of the type of illness you have, virtually any consultation with a physician will begin with a discussion of the history of your own general health and sometimes those of family members. The reason the doctor may ask you questions about parents, grandparents, or siblings is that some illnesses are genetically predisposed—they run in families.

Taking a good history is truly an art. Your doctor should take great care to ensure that you are as relaxed as possible. A good doctor will try to set you at ease by greeting you and shaking your hand as well as speaking in a calm, cheerful voice. Only when you feel comfortable with the physician and the situation in general will you be able to provide all the relevant information that your doctor needs. If you are anxious, you may forget something important or fail to listen attentively to the doctor's questions.

You may have discussed your case with many other individuals and possibly with some other physicians, and you may be absolutely convinced that you know what is really wrong with you. Nevertheless, when you go to your doctor's appointment, keep in mind that the doctor who is about to evaluate your problem is allowed no such luxury. A doctor who latches onto the first plausible diagnosis without considering other possibilities is not doing a good job. It's important to keep in mind one of the themes of this book: that low back pain has many different causes, including some that are life-threatening. For this reason, a doctor must consider a broad array of conditions during the initial consultation. Through your answers to many questions, findings from the physical exam, and possibly the results of paraclinical tests (such laboratory or diagnostic procedures as MRIs and electrophysiologic studies), the doctor will be able to reduce the number of possibilities and eventually make a solid diagnosis.

Questions to Expect

When the doctor first talks to you about the history of your back pain and your general health, you'll have your first opportunity to perceive any red flags that could lead you to consider consulting another practitioner. If a doctor fails to ask relevant questions, does not listen to your answers, or does not spend an adequate amount of time with you, seek help elsewhere. While it's true that few people die of low back pain, the failure to diagnose and treat this condition properly can lead to unnecessary suffering, not to mention unnecessary expense. Don't waste your time with someone who isn't enthusiastic about helping you.

During the questioning process, the physician should try to discern the pattern of your back pain—what seems to set it off, how long it lasts, what relieves it. The questions will also try to uncover other features of your condition that will enable the doctor to reject or confirm a possible diagnosis as economically as possible.

When did the pain start?   The doctor should try to identify the onset of your back pain. Has it been going on for weeks or months, or did it start yesterday? This is important for obvious reasons. If a patient was in an automobile accident the day before the back pain began, the diagnosis will differ significantly from the diagnosis for a patient who has experienced gradually worsening pain over a period of four to six weeks.

Do some actions make the pain worse?   The doctor should note any suggestion that your back pain is the mechanical type (the pain is worsened by movement). If this is so, he or she should ask you what particular types of movement exacerbate your pain. Because any of the small structural elements of the back can generate pain (not just the intervertebral discs, facet joints, and nerves), a doctor needs as much information as possible.

Do you have any symptoms involving your legs or bladder? A thorough, goal-oriented physician will be greatly interested in the presence of such symptoms. Pinched nerves in the back frequently cause severe low back discomfort that radiates into the legs. Although a pinched nerve isn't the only condition that can generate leg symptoms, the absence of leg symptoms makes the presence of a pinched nerve much less likely. Bladder symptoms might include pain in your bladder, difficulty with urination, or blood in your urine. A bladder or kidney infection can cause back pain.

Do you have pain in the thigh or buttock area?   Depending on the spinal level of the nerve involved, you may feel pain in the front of the thigh or through the buttocks, back of the thigh, and back of the calf. This pain is called sciatica because it goes along one of your sciatic nerves, the largest nerves in the body.

The presence of similar symptoms in both buttocks, thighs, or throughout your legs suggests that a relatively large structure is affecting your nerves. The doctor will consider the possibility of a large herniated disc or fairly severe lumbar stenosis. (Spinal stenosis, you may recall, is a narrowing of the canal that contains the spinal cord; so lumbar stenosis is a narrowing of this canal in the lumbar region.)

Do you have numbness in your legs?   If you do, don't wait for the doctor to ask this question. Numbness in one or both legs indicates that there may be pressure on a nerve and may motivate your doctor to do more testing, possibly ordering an MRI. Loss of sensation can impair the use of your limbs.

Do you have trouble moving your legs?   When a doctor considers whether your back problem may call for surgical treatment, weakness is commonly one of the determining factors. This is taken very seriously because leg weakness, even if fairly mild, can significantly affect your ability to walk and may lead to falls, difficulty exercising, and other problems. It is often permanent if neglected. (See chapter 8 to learn more about problems that require surgery.)

Are your bowels and bladder functioning normally? Herniated discs, lumbar stenosis, and some other low back conditions can affect the nerves that control the bowel and bladder. The symptoms, such as difficulty urinating or controlling bowel movements, are usually quite alarming and demand immediate medical evaluation.

When you change positions, does the pain change?   For example, does it improve when you lie down? Is it worse when you stand up? If your pain builds when you sit for a long time, the facet joints may be the source of your discomfort. Pain that isn't relieved by lying down can be serious; it may indicate an infection or even a tumor. (This is by no means always the case, however. We have seen patients with large herniated discs who insist they would rather stand than lie down, although we would think that a prone position would be far more comfortable.)

What other medical problems do you have?   You may believe that these problems have nothing to do with your back pain, but tell your doctor about them anyway. It's best to let him or her be the judge of whether any problems are related.

Do you have high blood pressure, coronary artery disease, or any other disease involving a major organ system? Have you ever experienced complications of atherosclerosis, such as stroke or chest pain?   The presence of hypertension, narrowed arteries, or a condition such as kidney disease or peptic ulcer disease will have a profound effect on the choice of medication. If you have ulcer disease, for example, nonsteroidal anti-inflammatory medications (NSAIDS) could trigger a "bleeding ulcer." Respond candidly to questions about other illnesses—you want your doctor to help you get better, not worse!

Are you allergic to any medications?   A doctor will certainly not want to prescribe any medicine that could give you a rash. Moreover, a severe allergic reaction can be life-threatening.

Do you smoke? Do you drink alcohol regularly?   Be honest. The doctor needs to consider any habits that affect your health. Smoking is a well recognized risk factor for degenerative disc disease, and excessive alcohol use can damage important organs, such as your liver, as well as cause your bones to lose important minerals.

Does your job require heavy lifting, or are you mostly sedentary at work? Are repetitive motions part of doing your job?   If you are employed, the doctor will want a detailed work history. It's important to the diagnosis and treatment for your doctor to know what kind of job you have and how you perform it.

Some of the questions the doctor asks will depend on whether you are male or female as well as how old you are. Your doctor is not being sexist or ageist. Some problems affect one sex more than the other or tend to develop more in older people than in younger ones.

If, for example, a woman is elderly or has a history of fractures in the wrists, spine, or hip, a doctor should give major consideration to the possibility of osteoporosis. The physician should ask the woman whether her mother has (or had) osteoporosis or any of its symptoms, such as hip or wrist fractures or a severely hunched back, since a tendency to develop this condition may be hereditary. Questions about whether a woman went through early menopause or has had hormone therapy should not be viewed as intrusive. The doctor must ask them to make the right diagnosis, because the answers have important implications about bone density, which relates to the health of your back.

We couldn't possibly list all the questions that a physician might pose to a patient with low back pain, but these are some of the basic ones. As the doctor takes your history, he or she will tailor the questions to your situation, taking into account such factors as the presence of trauma, your sex, your age, and how you characterize your pain.

Once the doctor thoroughly understands your complaint, he or she will form various hypotheses about its cause. The physical examination and subsequent tests will help the doctor to rule out some of these hypotheses until one diagnosis appears most likely.

The Physical Exam

After taking the history of your back pain and general health, the doctor will perform a physical examination of the lumbosacral spine (the lumbar and sacral regions of your back). Before the exam can begin, you must remove your clothes. A doctor cannot perform a complete physical examination on a fully dressed patient. We let patients keep their underwear on and provide a loose-fitting, adjustable gown for them to wear.

The exam process will allow your doctor to eliminate some of the items on his or her mental list of conditions that might be either directly responsible for your pain or contributing to it. The physician must assess your body's neurologic function, which refers to your general strength and your ability to perceive sensation. In addition, he or she will attempt to identify the actual source of your pain through various types of maneuvers. The doctor will ask you to move in different ways and will carefully observe your responses to see what motions cause more or less pain. As with the questions that help the doctor to form your history, the sequence of the various components of the examination is less important than the thoroughness of the physician's work.

A close inspection of the spine is usually the first step in the physical examination. Various types of congenital abnormalities (unusual conditions acquired during prenatal development) may not be readily apparent until later in life. For example, spina bifida occulta, a congenital abnormality in which the spine fails to complete its bony ring, is often accompanied by changes in skin coloration or by abnormal hair growth. Spondylolisthesis, in which part of the bony spine is fractured, frequently leads to very tight hamstrings (the muscles at the back of the thigh); this can give rise to an abnormal stance in which the knees are slightly bent.

The level of contraction of the paraspinal muscles (the muscles on either side of the bony spine) can influence the curvature of the low back. Muscle spasm (involuntary contraction usually caused by pain) on both sides may reduce the normal lumbar curve toward the front of the body, while spondylolisthesis can make this curve even more pronounced. Intense spasm on just one side of the spine can make the low back area bend visibly to that side.

After this inspection of your back, the doctor will usually test your spine's ability to move in various directions. To a certain degree, a healthy back can rotate and bend to either side, but most motion of the low back involves forward and backward bending. The doctor will note both the extent of your ability to move in these ways and also any increases in pain that result from the movements.

Symptoms related to facet joints are frequently worsened by overstretching the back, or backward hyperextension. The lumbar lordosis (natural curve toward the front of the body) should disappear as you flex. If this doesn't happen, a structural abnormality or internal ailment may be affecting the lumbar spine.

After the motion testing, the portion of the exam called palpation begins. To understand this word, remember that something is *palpable* if you can touch or feel it. Thus, during palpation, the physician will place his or her hands on your spine. The doctor will feel the spinous processes, which, as discussed in chapter 2, are the bony projections down the middle of the spine. Normally these points line up in a regular and even manner, but occasionally the doctor will find a "step"—a failure of the spinal processes to line up evenly—which suggests the possible presence of a fracture.

The doctor will also probe the paraspinal muscles and the facet joints (where one bony spine structure interlocks with another) in their flexed as well as extended positions, and he or she will identify and record the presence of trigger points (local, circumscribed areas of muscle spasm) or other areas of particular tenderness. With the palm of the hand, the doctor will firmly press and/or softly tap the midline structures.

"Percussion tenderness" suggests the possible presence of inflammation or even a malignant tumor in the tender area. The precise meaning of this finding is not immediately clear, however, and further maneuvers and tests will be required before a diagnosis can be made.

For example, most doctors use the straight-leg-raising test to aid the diagnosis of low back pain. In this very simple test, you lie on your back and then raise your legs one at a time. This movement stretches the lower lumbar nerve roots.

Although this test is not foolproof, if you have trouble holding your leg straight, one of these nerve roots may very well be inflamed.

The upper lumbar nerve roots can be tested in a similar manner: Lying on your abdomen, you bend each leg at the knee (or the doctor manipulates your leg for you); you then lift it as high as you can tolerate. Again, a radiating discomfort in the leg suggests that these nerve roots may be injured.

Just as we couldn't list every question that a doctor might ask you, we can't possibly discuss all the maneuvers a doctor might perform. But the preceding descriptions give you an idea of what to expect.

After the doctor has accomplished the leg maneuver tests, the actual neurological assessment can be undertaken. This usually begins with the doctor inspecting your muscles. Why? Because atrophy (the wasting away of muscles) commonly occurs when there are injuries to nerve roots. This atrophy is typically associated with demonstrable weakness. Keep in mind, however, that atrophy takes several weeks to occur and it's possible for a muscle to be profoundly weak and yet have normal bulk.

Your doctor will generally test your motor strength by having you move against resistance. For example, the doctor may ask you to push against his or her hand. This is an important test because the presence of significant muscle weakness is often one of the determining factors in the decision to treat a low back condition through surgery. An inexperienced examiner may have trouble detecting mild weakness, so it's crucial that your doctor is familiar with this condition in all its gradations.

The doctor may next test your reflexes. With a small hammer, the physician will tap various tendons, most commonly below the patella (for the knee-jerk response) and immediately above the heel (the so-called ankle jerk). Reflexes can also be checked by tapping tendons behind the knee joint. In the presence of radiculopathy (a pinched nerve in the back), the relative reflexes can be lost or diminished.

The doctor may also test your ability to perceive various types of sensation, possibly using a pinprick, a wisp of cotton or tissue, and a tuning fork. Your pattern of response will provide important information about your injury. For example, in a form of nerve root injury, the typical findings would include weakness and atrophy of the front thigh muscles (quadriceps) along with a reduced knee jerk and a loss of sensation on the inside of the knee.

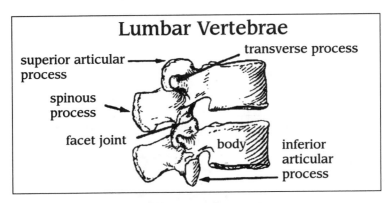

Figure 4-1 In a normal bone structure, two levels of the low back spine join together.

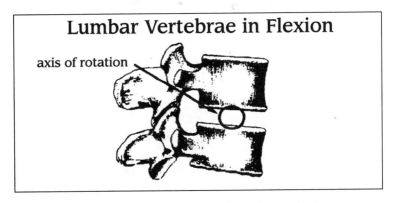

Figure 4-2 When the spine is flexed (bent forward), the rotational axis is located at the middle of the intervertebral disc.

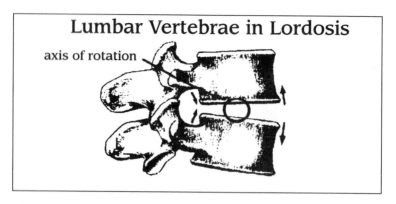

Figure 4-3 When the spine is arched, the rotational axis remains at the middle of the intervertebral disc.

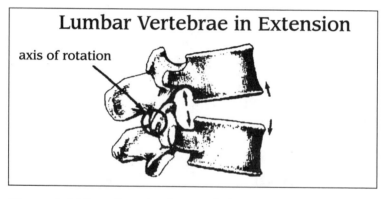

Figure 4-4 When the spine is extended too far back, the facet joint can be irritated.

In another form of nerve root injury, the typical findings would include atrophy of the muscles at the back and front of the thigh, as well as difficulty lifting the ankle upward. Sensory loss would be noted on the top of the foot and on the outer side of the calf.

Finally, there's the rectal examination. No one enjoys having this exam, but it may be necessary to evaluate your condition. Why? Because a rectal exam is frequently a useful tool in the diagnosis of lumbosacral conditions, and it's the only way for a doctor to examine the inside of the sacrum and to assess the rectum's ability to contract.

Once again, we have discussed only the most commonly used examination procedures because there are simply too many for us to explain them all. Your doctor may do other types of diagnostic testing during the physical exam. If you don't understand what he or she is doing (or why), be sure to ask.

Tests Your Doctor May Order

In many cases, your doctor may order additional tests whose results will help to analyze your condition. We will now explain many of the tests used in evaluating low back pain, starting with the most commonly used.

X-Rays

The x-ray technique has been used for more than a century. It is simple, quick, and quite reliable for detecting many spinal disorders. When performed in the context of a thorough physical exam and an accurate personal history, it is frequently the only necessary test for diagnosis.

The x-ray technician generally takes five views of the lumbar spine. These include an anterior-posterior view (front to back), a lateral view (side), two oblique (slantwise) views, and a specific lateral view of the lumbosacral junction. The oblique views show the bony opening through which the nerve roots exit. Additional views may supplement these five. In particular, flexion (bent over) and extension (bent backward) views may be helpful.

So, what can we learn from x-rays? Frequently plain x-rays of the lumbar spine are useful after fractures. The x-rays are quite sensitive for demonstrating fractures, though X-ray interpreters do occasionally miss small fractures. Nevertheless, as a general rule, the structural and weight-bearing integrity of the spine can be accurately assessed with x-rays.

Furthermore, bone spurs, which an MRI scan may miss, can often be detected with x-rays, particularly in the oblique views. Also detectable through x-rays is spondylolisthesis, a condition in which the vertebral bodies have separated from the bony arches of the vertebrae. Flexion and extension views of the lumbar spine are frequently helpful in detecting this particular condition. Diagnosis is very important because spondylolisthesis can be associated with abnormal and potentially hazardous movements of the vertebrae.

Although x-ray imaging does not clearly show the intervertebral discs, a radiologist can often reach some tentative conclusions about the state of an intervertebral disc from the height of the space between two adjacent vertebral bodies.

Doctors may also use simple x-ray techniques to identify bone cancer, osteoporosis, and various other conditions. In short, this technique is quick, useful, and less expensive than many other tests, but it does expose the patient to radiation and frequently misses conditions more readily diagnosed through other imaging studies.

Magnetic Resonance Imaging (MRI)

Magnetic resonance imaging, formerly called nuclear magnetic resonance imaging, is an exciting and fairly recent technique that doctors use to diagnose low back problems. It produces a very good computerized image of the intervertebral discs and the nerve roots. The test works through magnetic fields that alter the orientation of molecules in the body's tissues.

Although MRI may fail to detect some bony abnormalities, the images of the discs and nerves are quite excellent. Like an x-ray, an MRI is entirely painless, but unlike an x-ray, no exposure to radiation occurs. In addition, by altering the technique, the MRI technician can obtain images that emphasize different portions of the anatomy.

The MRI is the logical choice for most back pain cases in which an additional study is required after x-rays are taken. An MRI can be done after the patient receives contrast material, an intravenous injection that shows up clearly in the MRI. Contrast material will frequently appear in excessive amounts in abnormal tissue processes—for example, scar tissue that has developed after surgery. Furthermore, MRI is the most sensitive method for identifying cancer in the bony portions of the spine.

An MRI is expensive, costing an average of $1,200 in 1995. Patients may object not only to the cost of the MRI but also to being confined in very tight quarters during the scan, which usually takes from thirty to forty-five minutes. Although some patients feel claustrophobic in the small chamber used for MRIs, this may be remedied with the use of a mild tranquilizer. Recently developed scanners have made significant advances with regard to this confinement by providing a more open chamber in which the patient is unlikely to feel panicky. One remaining problem with MRIs is that they cannot be performed on patients with certain types of artificial heart valves, pacemakers, or metal clips placed during previous surgery.

Myelography

Myelography is a procedure in which dye is injected through the dural sac (the fluid-filled sac surrounding the spinal cord) and x-rays are taken in various planes. Radiologists, neurosurgeons, orthopedic surgeons, and occasionally neurologists perform this test, which is analogous to a spinal tap, except that rather than fluid being removed, it is injected.

The injected dye gives the cerebrospinal fluid an opaque quality that makes it visible in x-rays. The fluid-filled space envelops the nerve roots, essentially like a sleeve. If this "sleeve" doesn't fill properly, then the doctor will suspect the presence of some type of compressive abnormality, such as a pinched nerve. Odd configurations or indentations in the large vertical column of dye also suggest the presence of a compressive abnormality.

This study is often followed by a CAT scan of the areas in question. The two tests together allow the physician to form a picture of the contrast between bone and nerve. Thus myelography is another powerful tool in the diagnosis of lumbar disease.

Computerized Axial Tomography (CAT)

The CAT scan is another useful technique in the diagnosis of lumbar disorders. This test produces a cross-sectional image of the body's internal structures by computerized manipulation of x-rays.

Computerized axial tomography is the most accurate technique currently available for detecting bone spurs and fractures. In addition, it is the premier method for examining a cross-section of the spinal canal. For this reason, the CAT scan is a very effective tool in the diagnosis of lumbar stenosis (narrowing of the spinal canal in the lumbar region). Computerized tomography also produces a fairly accurate image of the intervertebral discs.

A single CAT scan usually takes much less time than an MRI scan; hence the CAT image tends to be less distorted from the patient's movement. Also, as a general rule, the patient feels less cramped in the CAT scanner. Another advantage is that people with cardiac pacemakers and similar devices may have these scans.

Electrophysiologic Tests

The previously described tests produce images, providing the clinician with visual information about the patient's anatomy. Other types of tests can shed light on how particular structures are working. Electrophysiologic testing gives us information about how nerves are functioning.

Electromyography is one kind of electrophysiologic study. The electromyogram, or EMG, is actually a two-part test. The first portion examines nerve conduction in a part of the body—in this case, the legs. This nerve conduction study can be performed on sensory as well as motor nerves. (Sensory nerves carry impulses from the sense organs to the nerve centers; motor nerves carry impulses that cause movement in the muscles.)

Electrodes are placed on the skin over sensory nerves, or on the skin above individual muscles. After the sensory or motor nerve is stimulated, an oscilloscope records the surface potential (change in electric state). By stimulating the nerves at various distances from the point of recording, the speed of impulse conduction in the nerve is calculated. The size of the potential that is measured gives some indication of how efficiently the nerve transmits an impulse. In very simple terms, this suggests how well (or how poorly) a nerve conducts electricity.

The second portion of this study is the EMG proper. In this procedure, a needle with a recording electrode is placed into a muscle. An oscilloscopic recording of the muscle is obtained during rest and during activity. Abnormalities recorded on the oscilloscope suggest how well the nerve that supplies the muscle can function.

What does all of this mean? Numbness, weakness, other dysfunction, or pain in the legs can be caused by pinched nerves in the back, but these symptoms may also result from generalized nerve disorder or nerves that are trapped at sites outside of the immediate spinal area.

The EMG will help to locate the problem affecting the nerves. A normal EMG strongly indicates that there is no major nerve injury in the spine or elsewhere along the course of the nerves to the legs.

Another electrophysiologic study used to diagnose low back disorders is the evoked potential, or the somatosensory evoked potential. Like the EMG, this study involves stimulating nerves in the legs, but it can also be performed in the arms.

In this test, either a specific nerve or a specific area of skin supplied by a nerve root is stimulated. Responses are recorded at various sites along the course of the nerve, at the spinal cord, and, frequently, at the brain level as well.

The somatosensory evoked potential is fairly difficult to perform correctly, and the procedure is fraught with technical problems. It has many advocates, however, and some studies indicate that it's one of the most sensitive techniques for identifying the presence of a pinched nerve.

Bone Scans

Bone scans have been in clinical use for decades. This test involves the administration of a radioactive isotope, which will collect in greater amounts in areas of abnormal bone. Inflammation, infection, and cancer will typically cause increased concentration of the radioactive isotope. A bone scan can be performed on specific sections of the body as well as over the entire skeletal system, making it a very useful screening technique.

When an individual with a history of cancer develops pain in the low back or other bony areas, his or her doctor is likely to order a bone scan. This test is probably less sensitive than MRI in detecting bony cancer. However, it can, as noted, allow examination of the entire skeleton rather than only a specific portion.

Keep in mind that a bone scan does expose you to radiation (though it is a minimal amount). Moreover, the procedure requires you to lie flat for an hour or even longer, which can be tough when your back is already making you uncomfortable. The scan of the entire skeleton generally lasts four hours.

Ultrasonography

Ultrasound uses high-frequency vibrations to form an image of internal body structures and thus detect abnormalities or injuries. While ultrasound technology is frequently used to diagnose abdominal and blood vessel disease, it can also be a valuable diagnostic tool in the evaluation of patients with low back pain. The primary object is to identify areas of inflammation that the doctor may be unable to see or feel.

Ultrasonography has proved useful in detecting conditions that affect the shoulder and other joints. Yet its role in evaluating low back pain syndrome is far from clear. Furthermore, the technique is very demanding in a technical sense; only the results produced by an experienced technician can be considered valid.

Thermography

This test evaluates heat emission from the skin. The patient removes his or her clothes and stands in a cool room before a heat sensor. Typically, three periods of heat emission are recorded and then considered by the interpreting physician.

Proponents of this technique claim that the thermal pattern can help with diagnosing back pain syndrome and will identify the presence of a nerve root injury or show whether the joints of the spine or supporting muscles are involved in the problem. But as with many diagnostic studies (as well as therapies for managing low back pain), thermography is not clearly supported by medical research. Further scientific investigation is needed to determine its usefulness.

In our own practice, we rarely use this type of study to evaluate patients with low back syndrome, but we do use thermography to diagnose reflex sympathetic dystrophy, a painful and enigmatic condition that usually occurs after trauma to a limb.

Discogram

In this test, a special opaque dye is injected into an intervertebral disc. (This substance appears bright on x-rays.) Proponents of this procedure feel that the distribution of the injected material and its absorption can produce some useful information about how much the intervertebral disc has degenerated.

The injection of the material occasionally causes the patient's symptoms to recur, which is conceivably a useful diagnostic indicator for what is actually causing the pain. Occasionally cortisone and novocaine are injected, both to reduce the pain and to aid diagnosis.

While discograms are frequently performed at research centers, they are not readily available at most hospitals. We do not use this procedure in our clinical practice. In fact, the reasons for performing it are unclear. One situation in which it might be helpful, in our view, is if someone has a clear history of sciatica but imaging studies have failed to indicate the abnormalities that are causing it; a discogram could conceivably help to identify the source of this person's pain. There's no doubt that more will be written on this subject in the future.

Conclusion

When diagnosing problems related to the lumbar spine, the modern clinician has many sophisticated tools available. However, the intelligent doctor will rely most heavily on the patient's history and on a careful physical examination because these provide the most reliable and cost-effective sources of information. The doctor will then choose the tests that are most likely to reveal any conditions that may be present. Going about the diagnosis in this way will efficiently pinpoint the cause of the problem as well as minimize the patient's discomfort.

To summarize, the doctor you see should spend plenty of time with you during your first appointment (as much as thirty minutes), first asking questions and listening carefully to your answers, and then examining your body—your bones, your muscles, how you move, where you hurt. After this process, your doctor should carefully select any further tests to help uncover what is wrong. In most cases, your physician will be able to select the one or two procedures that will determine the cause of your pain and lead to a correct choice of treatment. And, it is hoped, this treatment will lead to greatly diminished pain—perhaps even a pain-free existence—and a happier, more productive life.

5

Improving Your Back Through Simple Exercises

———∽∿∿∿∼———

When did it become okay to stop exercising? When you were ten? When you were twenty? When you were thirty-five? Maybe when you were fifty-five? Regardless of when regular exercise stopped being a part of your life, the correct answer to this question is: "It is never okay to stop exercising."

Exercise is not only the true fountain of youth, but it also prevents a significant source of acute and chronic back pain: weak back muscles. Without exercise, strong muscles become weak and already weak muscles become weaker. This leads almost inevitably to a painful back condition.

Heal Thyself

At our practice, Dr. Sudderth was fortunate to treat a medical colleague, a general practitioner who had been troubled by nagging back pain for some time. A very athletic man, he was involved in many sports and particularly fond of basketball.

He was accustomed to having discomfort in the low back, but when the feeling began to radiate into his legs, he finally realized that he couldn't continue to dismiss it as merely "back strain."

Doctors, nurses, and doctors' family members are notoriously difficult patients because, with their medical knowledge, they constantly second-guess their own physicians on both diagnosis and treatment. But this man was a surprisingly good patient, willing to provide needed information, ready to listen to advice, and committed to the process of getting well. Dr. Sudderth took a comprehensive history, did a thorough physical examination, and ultimately ordered an MRI. The scan revealed a bulging intervertebral disc.

As a family practitioner, this patient had prescribed exercises for many of his own patients, and now Dr. Sudderth instructed him to undertake a formal exercise program. The recommended regimen began with a warm-up, continued with stretching exercises for flexibility, and then concentrated on strength building. Even though the patient was already physically active, some areas of his body weren't receiving the workout they needed. A well-planned exercise program corrected this.

The program worked well. In time, the patient/doctor was able to resume all of his previous activities. He now rides his bicycle to the office, is able to enjoy social events, and is back to his full work schedule. Moreover, he's no longer hampered by persistent back and leg pain.

This story goes to show that even individuals who basically know what to do sometimes need a little specific education and encouragement. In this case, the patient's recreational activities exercised his arms and legs and even gave his heart and lungs a good workout, but these sports failed to exercise adequately the small muscles of his low back (the supporting structures of the spine). With all his athletic endeavors, these back muscles gave out, and the result was low back pain.

The Lowdown on the Low Back

In most individuals with adequate trunk strength, the spine is able to withstand a great deal of pressure from weight, particularly as the body is carried with the assistance of the spinal column. In fact, you carry not just your own body weight, but your weight multiplied by the force of gravity, and this is the total force that your spine has to withstand. As you can imagine, especially in hefty individuals, this is a significant force.

The stronger the low back muscles, the more force the spinal column can adequately resist, both during an isolated act, such as lifting a heavy box, and during a repetitive activity, such as running. In addition, when the muscles are fit and toned, they fatigue less quickly. This ability to endure allows them to perform more repetitions of an activity; that is, if you've built up your muscles' endurance, you can run farther, climb up and down a ladder more times, play with your children longer, or even mop more floors without your back beginning to ache.

A study published in the *Journal of Clinical Orthopedics and Related Research* found that some of the smallest muscles are responsible for most of the spine's movements that lead to extending or arching the back. This certainly explains why such stress is placed on these small back muscles.

In the work environment, people who have weak back muscles—particularly those whose activities require repetitive bending, twisting, or turning—suffer a significantly higher rate of back injury. But it's important to realize that individuals whose jobs involve physical labor are not the only ones at risk for back problems. People who maintain a bent posture while working, such as those who lean over drawing boards and those who sit for prolonged periods of time at their computers, are also at risk for developing back pain. A bent position seems to increase the pressure along the spinal column, as well as strain the back muscles.

Strong, flexible low back muscles are more able to resist not only acute injuries but also injuries that can develop and worsen over a long period of time. So even if your job demands little physical activity, well-maintained back muscles are extremely important.

But there are other important qualities of the low back muscles in addition to strength. Endurance, as previously mentioned, plays an important role in preventing injury to the low back muscles. Individuals with poor endurance in these muscles cannot maintain a single posture—whether it's standing, bending, sitting, or another position—for more than a short period of time without becoming tired. And muscle fatigue, due to a lack of endurance, is also a risk factor for developing low back pain. Combined with a loss of muscular flexibility, this lack of endurance can contribute significantly to back discomfort.

The Role of Age

A study that compared back muscle strength in various age groups, published in the *Journal of Spinal Disorders,* showed that individuals as young as twenty-one can show signs of moderate to marked degeneration of extensor strength in the low back muscles. Left unattended, the condition will not improve, because muscle function and strength deteriorate progressively as individuals age.

From the ages of twenty to forty, these muscles actually change very little. But from age forty-one through age sixty, muscle strength slowly and steadily declines, with more than 75 percent of individuals over the age of sixty having some degree of moderate or severe degeneration.

It is important to keep in mind, however, that weakened trunk muscles rarely occur by themselves. Instead, they are typically accompanied by other ailments. Degenerative joint changes, degenerative disc disease, facet syndrome (inflammation of the joints between the vertebrae), or another condition typically contributes to the decline in strength of the low back muscles.

The Role of the Abdomen

Patients frequently ask us, "Will it help my back if I do stomach exercises, such as sit-ups?" We respond by pointing out that most patients do not have back pain because of weakened abdominal muscles, but rather because of weakened low back muscles. It is therefore essential to address the fundamental problem, which is the weak back.

The Role of Inactivity

This brings us to another significant process, the deconditioned low back, or "chronic disuse atrophy." Basically, this state occurs when a person who has back pain, either from trauma or an injury that developed gradually, uses the back muscles even less frequently because of the pain. As he or she no longer uses these muscles, their strength decreases. In addition, with disuse, the ligaments, tendons, and joints become stiff. Too many people get caught up in this negative spiral.

The problem is that the ligaments, tendons, joints, and muscles are less able to avoid further injury. They are also ill prepared for the stresses of everyday living. Bending, standing, walking, lifting, twisting, and sitting can become quite painful. Ordinary activities can lead to additional injury, which, of course, leads to additional pain. As you can see, this weakened state puts a vicious cycle in motion.

We can sum up the cycle this way: pain; avoidance of activity; weakened muscles and supporting structures; reinjury; more pain. This is a critical concept when it comes to understanding chronic low back pain. If you perceive the role of deconditioning, you will grasp the importance of breaking out of this painful cycle.

Risk Factors for Low Back Pain

According to Dr. Kirkaldy-Willis, the major factors that contribute to back pain include:

1. Decreased fitness
2. Smoking
3. Weak trunk strength
4. Obesity
5. Stress
6. Depression
7. Alcohol or drug abuse
8. Psychosocial problems

As you can see, a significant factor in developing low back pain is a lack of trunk strength. The way to prevent or fix this problem is exercise, which we will soon discuss in detail. Regular, correctly performed exercise is what ends the chronic disuse atrophy syndrome, but exercise also plays a role in improving psychological health, in raising the pain threshold, and, of course, in enhancing general fitness.

All About Exercise

We all know that exercise does good things for our bodies and our minds. So why don't we do it? As physicians who have treated painful spine conditions for many years, we have heard almost every excuse you might come up with. Do you recognize any of these?

- It's too hot outside.
- It's too cold outside.
- It's raining.
- It's too sunny.

- I don't have the right equipment.
- I don't have the right workout clothes.
- I don't have the money to join a gym.
- I'll do it later/tomorrow/next week/next month.
- It will make my blood pressure worse.
- It will hurt my heart.
- I'm too old.

Patients have told us that they can't exercise because of their arthritis, because of their lung conditions, because their diabetes will flare up, or because their diabetes is already too severe. We've heard the excuse that their knees hurt, their ankles hurt, or, of course, their backs hurt, and that's why they can't exercise. Patients have explained to us that they simply don't know what exercises to do or that different doctors or physical therapists have given them conflicting exercises for their spine pain syndrome.

Whatever your explanation is for why you don't exercise, we can scientifically and convincingly refute it. When you perform appropriate exercises in a safe, effective, controlled fashion, a home exercise regimen or a directed program of exercise therapy should not prove a risk to your health. Instead, it will reduce your back pain, promote the healing of many other medical conditions, and enhance your general health.

It is simply no longer acceptable for a back pain patient to say, "I don't like to exercise." (Even if it's true.) With all the information available today on the value of exercise, and the many recent studies that have explored the best treatments for chronic back pain, no one can deny that exercise regimens are important in preventing and alleviating back pain.

Getting Started

Stop! Don't hoist that dumbbell over your head just because you're eager to strengthen your back and some other guy at your new gym is lifting heavy weights. Not every exercise is suited to every individual, and it's essential to devise an exercise program that is appropriate for your own body. Furthermore, any physical activity carries with it a risk of injury. Before starting a vigorous program, you should discuss specific exercises and plan your regimen with the physician who has examined your back and knows the history of your health.

We have one other caution for you: Remember that, as the saying goes, "Rome was not built in a day." Just as a bodybuilder slowly restructures and rebuilds his or her body over a period of months to years, a person with acute or chronic back pain will gradually strengthen weak muscles and lessen the pain. You need to realize that this is a slow, steady process, not a quick fix.

To begin your program, you do not need fancy athletic gear, membership in an expensive health club, or a personal trainer. You do need to be comfortable, however, with well-made athletic shoes that fit properly and absorbent, loose-fitting clothes. No longer do women wear only leotards; many exercise in T-shirts and shorts or cotton pants. So don't feel that your body needs to look perfect when you start working out at a local gym. On the other hand, don't wear anything bulky that might restrict your range of motion as you go through your exercise regimen. As for where you go to exercise, most areas have inexpensive fitness programs. Check with your local hospital to see whether it has a program.

Warming Up

Warming up your muscles is essential to preparing for increased activity and reducing the chance of injury. The warm-up will raise your body temperature, increase blood circulation, and help to improve muscle flexibility. Either an active warm-up, such as taking a brisk walk, or a passive warm-up, such as applying a heating pad, will loosen tightness in your back and get your whole body ready to work out.

To perform an active warm-up, maintain an activity for at least five to ten minutes. You can do this by walking (even walking in place), dancing, chair exercises, or marching in place—anything that gets you moving. If you have access to a stair-climbing machine, stationary bicycle, or treadmill, five to ten minutes on this equipment certainly works well for warming up your body.

If you haven't exercised regularly in the past and have experienced back pain for a long time, you may have a low level of physical endurance. It is perfectly acceptable to use a heating pad to warm your low back muscles before beginning a workout. Keep the heating pad, turned to its lowest setting, on the low back region for fifteen to twenty minutes. Another option is to rub a heating lotion into the low back area for thirty minutes; after this, the muscles should be warm and ready to be exercised.

Flexibility

This is the second element of a general fitness and strengthening program. Your work to improve flexibility should follow your warm-up activities. Begin with simple stretches, moving slowly and paying attention to how your body responds. The goal of flexibility training is to increase the range of motion in your joints to a level that will protect a joint and its surrounding tissues from injury.

The following guidelines will help you to stretch safely and effectively:

1. Begin by moving gently into the starting position.
2. Take several slow, deep breaths to help yourself relax.
3. Exhale slowly as you move into the stretch.
4. Stop at the point of discomfort and before you feel pain.
5. Hold the position for ten to twenty seconds, breathing normally.
6. Take another deep breath, and slightly ease off the stretch.
7. Exhale as you move deeper into the stretch, and hold.

8. Repeat steps 5 through 7 as often as you can and as time allows.

Stretching movements must be performed in a slow, controlled, and steady manner. Many people try to increase their flexibility by bouncing while in a stretch position, but this is a very bad idea, as it can lead to muscle tears. Never try to jiggle yourself into position. Furthermore, doing exercises too rapidly or bouncing can give you too much momentum, when what you really need to do is stretch your muscles.

Also, be aware that flexibility increases slowly. You'll find that it takes from three to twelve weeks to notice a difference, so be patient. It may help to keep this in mind: If you do not do these warm-up and stretching exercises, and twelve weeks go by, you have lost twelve weeks. If, on the other hand, you do the exercises, and twelve weeks go by, you have almost certainly increased the function and flexibility of your muscles as well as the range of motion in your joints, and you have lost nothing in the meantime.

Strength Training

You should do the strength-training exercises three to four times a week. The goal here is to build strength in the soft tissues that support and stabilize the spine, the pelvis, and the trunk. Before beginning your strength-building activities, however, you should establish your warm-up and flexibility program. Don't begin strength training until you have experienced an increase in your joints' range of motion. You will probably need to follow the stretching regimen for three to four weeks before you'll be ready to start on muscle strengthening.

These guidelines will make the strengthening segment work for you:

1. Always begin with the warm-up and appropriate stretches.

2. Begin each exercise with ten repetitions.

3. After you've worked up to two sets of twenty-five repetitions, add resistance (using soup cans, one- to two-pound weights, or plastic bags filled with sand or dirt).

4. Continue to increase the repetitions and resistance as the exercises become easier for you.

5. Repeat steps 1 through 4 until you have reached a weight load of five pounds.

Remember that exercises performed with improper technique or an excessive weight load will not speed the strengthening process. In fact, the muscle groups you want to build may end up injured, which will set back the entire strengthening process.

Be sure to follow our explanations and illustrations, checking them frequently until the correct positions and movements become second nature. In addition, keep in mind that strength is even slower to increase than flexibility. It may take three to twelve weeks, or even longer, before you become noticeably stronger. Therefore, as in all other aspects of exercise, patience is a virtue and persistence brings rewards.

For quick reference, here is the basic exercise schedule. Full descriptions of each exercise are given in the following section of this chapter. As you progress in the program, you will add the exercises for subsequent weeks to the exercises you are already doing (in other words, when you begin the plan for week two, you won't stop doing the exercises for week one).

Week 1

1. Back stretch
2. Calf, hip, and thigh stretches
3. Seated thigh stretch
4. Abdominal contraction with diaphragmatic breathing

Week Two

5. Side stretch
6. Bend and side stretch
7. Seated/lying hip and buttock stretch
8. Pelvic tilt
9. Lower trunk rotation

Week Three

10. Abdominal crunches
11. Passive trunk extension
12. 90-degree wall slides
13. Side bend
14. Wide-knee squats
15. Hip-wide squats
16. Knee extensions
17. Knee curls

An Illustrated Regimen

Everyone, including individuals who have never experienced low back pain, can benefit from the following exercise program. The exercises will help to correct problems that are associated with back pain. These problems are a result of poor spinal alignment or posture, improper body mechanics (including sitting incorrectly at a desk; poor sleeping position; and lifting, twisting, or bending incorrectly), repetitive movements, or simply being in poor physical shape.

Week One

1. *Back Stretch*

    Position   Sit at the edge of a chair, with your feet apart and your knees and ankles aligned. Make sure the chair is stable.

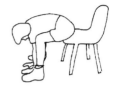

Movement Reach both hands toward the floor, relaxing your head and neck. Hold for 10–30 seconds.

Goal To place your palms on the floor. (This may not happen for a few days, weeks, or even months, so don't be discouraged and don't try to push beyond your physical limits.)

2. *Calf, Hip, and Thigh Stretches*

   Position Stand by a chair or a counter for support. Your feet should be shoulder-width apart, with one leg back and one leg forward. Stand tall, with your shoulders back and abdominals in. Check that your hips are square, your toes are pointing forward, and the forward knee is aligned with the ankle.

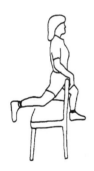

   Movement for the calf stretch Tuck the buttocks under, and straighten the knee that's behind you. Hold for 20–30 seconds. Repeat with the other leg.

   Movement for the hip stretch Place the knee on a chair (knee behind hip), and lean the hip forward. Hold for 20–30 seconds. Repeat with the other leg.

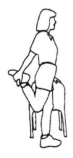

   Movement for the thigh stretch Grab the back foot and draw it toward the buttocks. Hold for 20–30 seconds. Repeat with the other leg.

   Modification Try this if you have trouble with the standard stretch: Hold onto a counter or chair for support. Place another chair behind you. Place one knee on the back chair and lean slightly forward until you feel a stretch.

Goals   To keep the knee behind the hip. To squeeze your buttocks and pull your hip forward.

3.   *Seated Thigh Stretch*

Note: This is a progressive stretch. Start with stage 1 until you no longer feel a stretch, then move into stage 2, and so on.

Position   Sit on the edge of a chair. One leg is bent at 90 degrees (knee right above ankle), and the other leg is straight out with the toe toward the ceiling. (Do not lock your knee.)

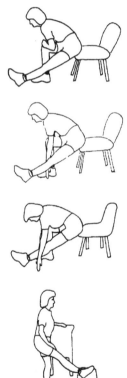

Movement for stage 1   Place both hands on the bent leg, and lean your chest toward the bent knee. Hold for 20–30 seconds. Repeat on the other side.

Movement for stage 2   Move both hands toward the floor, straddling your bent leg. Hold for 20–30 seconds. Repeat on the other side.

Movement for stage 3 Straddling the straight leg, place hands on the floor. Hold for 20–30 seconds. Repeat on the other side.

To advance   When you are comfortable with the third stage, try it with your toes rotated in, and then with them rotated out. Hold each position for 20–30 seconds.

Modification   Stand by a counter or chair for support, chest out and shoulder blades squeezing together. Place the heel of one foot on a stool, and push your tailbone backward. The supporting knee remains slightly bent. Hold for 15–20 seconds. Repeat on the other side.

4. *Abdominal Contraction with Diaphragmatic Breathing*

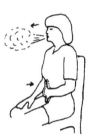

Position   Either lying with knees bent or sitting with back straight.

Movement   Pull your abdominals in toward your spine as you breathe out. Allow the abdominals to relax, or pouch out, as you breathe in. Do 15–25 repetitions. If you are doing this correctly, you will feel pressure in your lower back as you exhale.

Goal   To retrain the body to breathe correctly.

Week Two

5. *Side Stretch*

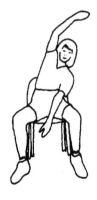

Position   Sit tall with both buttocks on a chair.

Movement   Reach your right arm up over your head while bending to the left and keeping your buttocks squarely on the chair. Reach up, over, and back as you pull your abdominals in. Do not let your right shoulder drop forward. Drop your left shoulder toward the floor. Hold for 15 seconds. Repeat on the other side.

6. *Bend and Side Stretch*

    Position   Sit on the edge of a chair, feet together and knees aligned with ankles.

    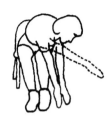

    Movement   Twist to one side, and both arms toward the floor (at your side). Hold for 15–20 seconds. Repeat on the other side.

    Modification   If you can't perform a full twist, begin by straddling your leg; gradually work toward a twist by walking your hands around.

    Goals   To place your hands on the floor and then reach your elbow toward your ear. To keep your shoulders parallel to the floor.

7. *Seated/Lying Hip and Buttock Stretch*

    Position   Sit tall with both buttocks on the chair. Place one ankle on the opposite thigh.

    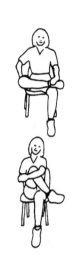

    Movement   Apply pressure to the crossed thigh. Hold for 15 seconds. Move the opposite shoulder toward the crossed knee as you hug the knee into your chest and toward the opposite shoulder. Hold for 15 seconds. Straighten your back, and hold for 5 seconds. Repeat on the other side.

    Goals   To keep your buttocks squarely on the chair. To sit tall with your back straight.

    Modification   If this stretch is too difficult for you, it can also be done lying on the floor.

    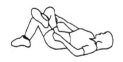

Position   Lie on your back with your knees bent. Place your ankle on the opposite knee.

Movement   Push your knee out by applying pressure to the crossed thigh. Hold for 15–30 seconds. Lift your shoulders off the floor, and hug the bent leg. Pull your foot off the floor as you move your knee toward your head (keep the thigh pressed out). Hold for 15 seconds. Repeat on the other side.

8. *Pelvic Tilt*

Position   Lie on the floor or another hard surface, feet flat and
knees bent.

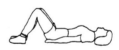

Movement   Breathe by pulling in
your abdominal muscles (see exercise 4). Use your back muscles
to flatten the lower back into the floor. Hold for
5 seconds, then relax. Do 25 repetitions.

Goal   To relax your buttocks and upper torso so that you only contract the lower trunk muscles.

9. *Lower Trunk Rotation*

Position   Lie on the floor or another hard surface, knees bent and
shoulders flat against the floor.

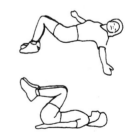

Movement for stage 1   Move both
knees to the side, and hold for 15
seconds. Come back to center, then
move to the opposite side and hold.

Movement for stage 2   Lift your
knees toward your chest, turn to
one side, and hold for 15 seconds.
Come back to center, then turn to
the opposite side and hold.

To advance   Apply pressure to the top knee, using the hand closest to your rotated knees. This will increase the stretch.

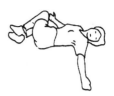

Hint   It's important to keep both shoulders on the floor.

Goal   To have your bent legs relaxed against the floor without the opposite shoulder rising.

Week Three

10. *Abdominal Crunches*

Position   Lie on the floor or another hard surface, feet flat and knees bent.

Movement   With your hands at your sides, perform the pelvic tilt and exhale (see exercise 8) as you lift your head and shoulders off the floor. Move your hands toward your ankles as you lift. Hold for 1–2 seconds, then release briefly as you relax and inhale. Build up to 2 sets of 25.

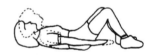

Hint   Your neck and head should be in a rigid position. Pretend to be holding an apple between your chin and chest while lifting.

Note   This is a small movement. Your shoulders should not lift more than 4–7 inches off the floor. Also, your neck should not feel strained; be sure your abdominal muscles are doing the work.

11. *Passive Trunk Extension*

> *Position*   Lie on your abdomen,
> arms bent at your sides.

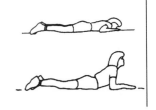

> *Movement*   Using your arms,
> slowly lift your torso. Support
> the torso with your elbows as
> you hold for 20–40 seconds.

> *Note*   You should feel your ab-
> dominal muscles stretching but
> should not feel strain in your low back. If you experience
> any pain, discontinue this exercise immediately.

12. *90-Degree Wall Slides*

> *Position*   Stand with your back against a wall; your feet
> should be 1–2 feet from the wall. Press your head and
> shoulders firmly against the wall, so that your upper body
> is correctly aligned. Check the alignment of your legs and
> feet, too; when you slide down the wall, your knees and
> ankles should be parallel.

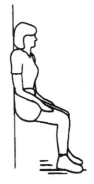

> *Movement*   Slide down the wall (mov-
> ing toward a sitting position but going
> only as far as you can tolerate), and
> then perform a strong pelvic tilt (see
> exercise 8). Hold for 15 seconds. Slide
> back up the wall. Repeat 10 times. (If
> your legs begin to shake, go only half
> as far down as you went at first.)

> *Hint*   Keep your tailbone on the wall
> as you flatten your back.

> *Note*   Follow this exercise with the back stretch and the
> calf, hip, and thigh stretches (exercises 1 and 2).

> *Goals*   To maintain the pelvic tilt and correct posture,
> feeling this in your lower abdomen. To have your

buttocks and knees on the same plane. To keep your head, shoulders, spine, and buttocks pressed firmly against the wall.

13. *Side Bend*

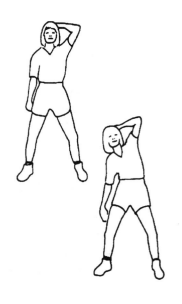

Position   Stand tall, knees slightly bent and feet about shoulder-width apart for good balance. Place your left hand on top of your head. Pull your shoulders back, and keep your lower body stationary. Look straight ahead.

Movement   Bend to the right until you feel a stretch along your left side. Pull your abdominals in, and forcefully exhale as you lift back to center. Do 10 repetitions.

Note   Follow this exercise with the abdominal contractions and the side stretch (exercises 4 and 5).

14. *Wide-Knee Squats*

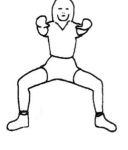

Position   Your feet should be more than shoulder-width apart, with your toes and knees pointed at a 45-degree angle and your arms extended for balance.

Movement   Move your body weight onto your heels as you sit back and down (you bend at the hip *and* the knees). Keep your back straight. As you lift, pull your abdominal muscles in and exhale.

Modification If you can't do this exercise because of instability, use a counter or door handle for balance. Try the freestanding squat again in 3 weeks.

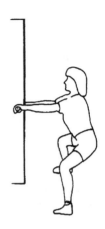

Hint If this squat causes discomfort, do the knee extensions and knee curls (exercises 16 and 17) for 3–6 weeks before trying squats again. These movements will strengthen your legs and help you to perform the wide-knee squat.

Note Follow the wide-knee squats with the back stretch and the calf, hip, and thigh stretches (exercises 1 and 2).

15. *Hip-Wide Squats*

Position Feet are hip-width apart, toes and knees pointing forward and arms extended for balance.

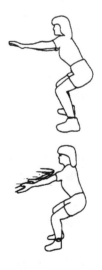

Movement Move your body weight onto your heels as you sit back and down (you bend at the hip *and* the knees). Keep your back straight. As you lift, pull your abdominals in and exhale.

Modification If you can't do this exercise because of instability, use a counter or door handle for balance. Try the freestanding squat again in 3 weeks.

Note Follow this exercise with the back stretch and the calf, hip, and thigh stretches (exercises 1 and 2).

16. *Knee Extensions*

Position for stage 1   Sit on a
chair with your back straight.

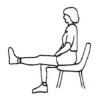

Movement for stage 1   Lift your
left foot approximately 1 inch off
the floor, then extend the left leg
until the knee is straight. (As you
straighten your leg, pull your abdominals in and exhale.) Hold
for 3–5 seconds, then slowly
bend your knee to return to the
starting position, with your foot
still 1 inch off the floor. Do not
rest your foot on the floor between repetitions. Do 10–25 repetitions. Repeat the exercise on
your right side.

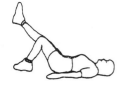

Position for stage 2   Lie on your back with your legs
together and knees bent. Make certain your knees stay
together.

Movement for stage 2   Straighten your left leg as you pull
in your abdominals and exhale. Bend your leg to return to
the starting position, but do not rest your foot on the
floor. Do 10–25 repetitions. Repeat the exercise on your
right side.

Note   Follow the knee extensions with the calf, hip, and
thigh stretches (exercise 2).

17. *Knee Curls*

Position   Lean your elbows on a counter or the back of a
chair, and tighten your abdominal muscles. Keep your
knees parallel, with one knee slightly behind the other
The supporting (forward) knee is slightly bent.

Movement   Lift your back foot up toward the buttocks, and hold for 1–2 seconds. Lower your foot, but do not rest it on the floor between repetitions. Do 10–25 repetitions. Repeat on the other side.

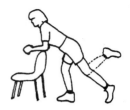

Note   Follow this exercise with the seated thigh stretch (exercise 3).

How You May Feel After Exercise

Now that we have outlined a home exercise regimen that will help you to increase your flexibility, endurance, and strength, we must point out that there is more to the picture than just doing the exercises.

You have doubtless heard the expression "No pain, no gain." In a limited sense, this is true, because a slight burning sensation in the muscles naturally occurs when you work them. However, you should never feel sharp or severe pain during an exercise; if you do, stop immediately and rest the area that hurts. We all know the difference between discomfort and pain. After exercising, you may have muscle inflammation and the associated discomfort, but you should not experience pain.

In fact, in the hours or days after a workout, your muscles may feel quite sore. Don't be discouraged by this, and don't let it keep you from exercising again. Think of the soreness as a positive sign that you have worked your muscles. You can also take some steps to relieve your pain.

Reducing the Pain That Follows a Workout

Many treatments will effectively reduce this muscle pain, which physicians refer to as myofascial pain. First of all, as we mentioned earlier in this chapter, you can prevent a good deal of postexercise pain by warming up the muscles prior to performing your exercises. You can do this with about ten minutes of a gentle aerobic activity, such as marching in place, or by applying a heating pad to the areas that get sore. After a stretching and strengthening workout, your options for reducing pain include having a therapeutic massage, a session of chiropractic care, or another kind of manipulative care. If you can't afford to see a professional, perhaps your partner or a close friend will give you a massage.

Many people aren't sure whether to apply cold or heat to sore muscles. During the acute phase (immediately after a workout), applying ice to the area of soreness may be helpful. If the soreness or stiffness persists, heat may then provide more comfort than cold.

Over-the-counter anti-inflammatory drugs (such as aspirin and ibuprofen), as well as over-the-counter nutritional supplements (such as vitamin E), can help with the muscle cramping and burning that may follow exercise. Vitamin C, as an antioxidant, is sometimes effective in reducing muscular pain, although its impact has not been as well documented as that of vitamin E therapy.

Whatever method you try, remember that in a short period of time the muscle pain from stretching, strengthening, and conditioning will decrease, while the positive results for which you're striving—increased range of motion, increased joint function, and, most importantly, increased low back strength—will appear and increase. When you begin to experience these positive results, the change will have a positive effect on your mood and motivation. You'll discover that the more you exercise, the better you feel, and this fact alone increases your tolerance for any lingering soreness. Feeling better is, after all, the ultimate goal.

6

Medications for Back Pain

At one time or another, you have probably taken some kind of medication to help you through an illness or injury. You may have had an infection for which your doctor prescribed antibiotics. Probably you have taken pain relievers for headaches and antacids for occasional stomach distress.

Most medications are prescribed on a temporary basis, though some must be taken every day for years or even a lifetime. In our practice, we frequently prescribe medications for patients with back complaints. Although we don't want them to be taking medicine for a long period of time, we recognize that a person who is in constant pain will usually not recover as quickly as a person whose pain is alleviated. Our goal, therefore, is to get the patient comfortable, initiate relevant therapy, and get him or her off the medication.

All medications can have side effects, even those that most people consider harmless. For example, acetaminophen—which you may know by its most common brand name, Tylenol—can have serious side effects if used on a prolonged basis or incorrectly.

In the United States, the most common medications used for pain are the nonsteroidal anti-inflammatory drugs (NSAIDs). The best-known of these is aspirin, but it is hardly the only option. More than twenty different NSAIDs are currently available for use by clinicians. In this large market, drug companies compete fiercely for their shares. You've probably noticed the numerous commercials for pain relievers that appear on television, and you may have felt unsure about which kind you should take for specific problems. In general, NSAIDs work to reduce inflammation, which is usually the cause of temporary aches and pains, as well as to relieve pain directly. This dulling of pain is called analgesia. A little later in this chapter, we will discuss specific analgesics and the differences among them.

Some of the medications usually used to alleviate low- to moderate-intensity pain are available on an over-the-counter basis. Unlike prescribed narcotics, most of these medications do not make you feel dazed or sleepy, although some of the longer-acting ones may do so. These over-the-counter drugs have certain side effects that may influence a person's ability to tolerate them.

Gastric irritation (stomach upset) is very common in this drug class and can even lead to life-threatening hemorrhage. This is particularly an issue with elderly patients and with patients on blood-thinning medication. To lessen the problem of stomach irritation, some NSAIDs are coated with substances that influence their absorption. Physicians often prescribe additional protective medications to reduce the risk of gastrointestinal side effects.

Another problem with NSAIDs is that they tend to reduce the flow of blood to the kidneys. For most people, this side effect may be inconsequential, but it can be quite dangerous for patients suffering from congestive heart failure, chronic kidney disease, or cirrhosis.

Keep in mind that these medications can also cause retention of fluid and salt, elevating the blood pressure and counteracting the effect of antihypertensive medications a person may be taking. If you know or suspect that you have high blood pressure, you should consult your doctor before choosing a pain reliever.

Other, less common side effects include rashes and liver damage. These can occur unpredictably in otherwise healthy individuals.

There is no single best pain reliever for everybody with back pain. You may respond well to one of the medications in this class and not respond as well to a different NSAID. And although an NSAID may relieve your pain, its side effects may be problematic. Hence your doctor may need to recommend or prescribe one pain reliever, discuss your response to this medicine with you after a few days, and then have you try a different pain reliever if you're unhappy with the first one. The doctor will base his or her choice of medication on efficacy, safety, tolerance, your willingness to take the medication in question, its cost, how easy it is to take, and how often you have to take it. Unfortunately, some of these medicines are not only very expensive but they are literally hard to swallow.

Discussing and analyzing all the medications on the market is beyond the scope of this book. But we will tell you something about the pain relievers that your doctor is most likely to recommend or prescribe for your back trouble. After reading this chapter, you will feel prepared to talk to your doctor about which analgesic might be best for you.

Commonly Used Medications

In this section, we discuss medicines that are frequently used to relieve back pain. These include both over-the-counter and prescribed drugs. Some of them will be familiar names, and others may be new to you.

Nonsteroidal Anti-Inflammatory Drugs (NSAIDs)

NSAIDs, as we stated earlier, lessen swelling and pain. Many of them are available without a prescription.

Aspirin   The first nonsteroidal anti-inflammatory drug, aspirin is very effective for most benign conditions that cause mild to moderate pain. According to some estimates, as much as 20,000 tons of aspirin are consumed in this country each year. That's a lot of aspirin!

An over-the-counter medication, aspirin usually must be taken every four hours, which some people find inconvenient. Children with viral infections should never be given aspirin because it can lead to the development of Reye's syndrome, a life-threatening illness. Aspirin is also a common cause of drug poisoning in children.

Aspirin reduces the blood's ability to clot and, for this reason, is often used in stroke prevention. However, this effect makes aspirin a bad choice for someone with an ulcer or another condition that involves bleeding. To reduce stomach irritation, coated aspirin is available, as are time-release and antacid formulas.

Ibuprofen   This enjoys a reputation among medical practitioners as a safe, effective, and low-cost NSAID. Ibuprofen is available both in prescription strengths and in over-the-counter preparations including Motrin, Advil, Nuprin, and Rufen. It can cause some gastrointestinal irritation, but less than does aspirin.

Cases of severe kidney damage as well as a noninfectious type of meningitis have been associated with the use of ibuprofen. But this is an extremely rare occurrence. People who take blood-thinning drugs should also be cautious about using ibuprofen. On the plus side, this medication has a very short half-life and is unlikely to accumulate in the body.

Ketoprofen   Oruvail, the brand name for the once-a-day, extended-release version of ketoprofen, is usually quite effective and very convenient for patients with chronic back pain. However, because it is released into the body gradually, Oruvail is not particularly effective at relieving acute pain. Ketoprofen is also available in a direct-release form (Orudis), which is now available over the counter.

Although this pill is taken just once a day, there is no risk of a poisonous buildup. The body eliminates ketoprofen much more quickly than it does the other once-a-day NSAIDs. This property is especially important for older patients.

Acetaminophen   Known mainly by the brand name Tylenol, acetaminophen does not actually belong to the NSAID class because it does not reduce inflammation. But it does have an analgesic effect and can be quite helpful for people with low back pain that is not extremely severe.

This medication lacks the gastrointestinal side effects of the anti-inflammatory medications. In fact, side effects from taking acetaminophen are relatively rare. High doses of acetaminophen, however, are known to cause liver damage, and extremely large doses can be lethal for this reason.

Acetaminophen is frequently formulated with other medications, including muscle relaxants and narcotics. When taken with a nonsteroidal anti-inflammatory medication, acetaminophen is probably more effective than when taken alone.

Naproxen Sodium   One of the most commonly used over-the-counter anti-inflammatory medications is naproxen sodium (prescription brand name Naprosyn), which has a reputation among doctors as a safe and effective choice. It is available in a low-cost generic alternative and recently became available without a prescription. (The common brand name for the over-the-counter version is Aleve.) Because this medication is taken only twice a day, many patients prefer it for its convenience.

Ketorolac   Marketed as Toradol, ketorolac is one of the newer arrivals on the nonsteroidal scene and has the advantage that it can be injected directly into the painful muscles. This is a fast-acting and very effective prescription NSAID. It's usually administered three to four times a day, for a short period only.

Diclofenac Sodium   This is another anti-inflammatory medication that your doctor may prescribe. The brand name is Voltaren. Typically taken twice daily, the pills are enteric coated to minimize stomach irritation (the enteric preparation means that they don't disintegrate until they reach the intestines).

In about 15 percent of the people taking diclofenac sodium, blood tests have revealed abnormal liver function. Patients should therefore have their blood tested eight weeks after beginning to take this medication.

Diclofenac sodium can interfere with the workings of both digoxin, a commonly used heart medication, and lithium, which is used to treat patients with manic-depressive disorder. A similar formulation, diclofenac potassium (brand name Cataflam), is now available for use in this country. Its advantage over diclofenac sodium is unclear.

Nabumetone   Another anti-inflammatory medication that doctors commonly prescribe is nabumetone (brand name Relafen). It has the reputation of being easier on the gastrointestinal system than its competitors.

While the risk of bleeding in the digestive tract appears to be diminished with nabumetone, it seems to have the same unpleasant gastrointestinal side effects as the other NSAIDs. These can include diarrhea and abdominal discomfort.

Oxaprozin   A relatively new nonsteroidal painkiller in this country, oxaprozin (brand name Daypro) appears to be quite effective and is taken in a convenient, once-a-day dosage. The body eliminates it steadily but slowly, creating the possibility of accumulation, especially in elderly patients. However, we have not observed this in our practice, in which we see predominantly older individuals. Note that if you are taking metoprolol (Lopressor), you should not take oxaprozin, as it may lead to an increase in blood pressure.

We have found that oxaprozin works well for many of our back pain patients. It effectively treats not only the soft tissue irritation, but also the inflammation of the facet joints.

Narcotics

The term *narcotic* comes from the Greek word *narkos,* which means "to numb." Narcotics are also known as opioid analgesics. *Opioid* refers to opiates, which are chemicals derived from morphine. While morphine itself is rarely used to treat back pain syndromes, other synthetic narcotic medications are frequently administered.

The use of opioid analgesics is one of the more controversial issues confronting doctors who treat low back conditions. Some physicians categorically refuse to prescribe narcotics even if a patient is in excruciating pain. We find this approach reprehensible. In our own practice, we use narcotics judiciously for the appropriate patients.

An oft-cited 1994 study by the U.S. Department of Health and Human Services, "Acute Low Back Problems in Adults," has suggested that while opioid analgesics can be helpful in the treatment of low back pain for a brief period of time, they appear to be no more effective in alleviating back symptoms than nonsteriodal anti-inflammatory medications or acetaminophen. The study goes on to identify various side effects of the opioids in use, including impaired judgment and drowsiness.

We take great issue with the study's conclusions about the efficacy of narcotics. Based on our personal observations in the treatment of thousands of patients with low back pain, we feel that narcotics are sometimes the best choice for pain relief, depending on the individual case.

While we agree that use of these medications can have significant side effects and even lead to addiction, we feel that narcotics are an important adjunct in the treatment of both patients with acute low back pain and patients with severely exacerbated chronic low back pain. We are aware that narcotics are frequently used improperly, but we refuse to "throw the baby out with the bathwater."

Side effects of narcotic analgesics include dizziness, fatigue, impaired concentration, blurred vision, and nausea. Particularly with the use of codeine, constipation is another major problem. Some of these medications, such as meperidine hydrochloride (brand name Demerol), are usually given by injection, while others are available in pill form. The oral medications frequently also include aspirin or acetaminophen. Examples are codeine, propoxyphene (Darvocet), oxycodone (Percocet), and hydrocodone (Lorcet).

Tramadol hydrochlorothide (brand name Ultram) is a recent arrival to this class of medication. This is a particularly exciting option because it appears to be as effective at relieving pain as the traditional opioids but without their high risk of chemical dependency.

Tramadol hydrochlorothide is actually a very weak opioid analgesic, but it has other properties that appear to interfere with pain sensation via neurotransmitters (substances that carry chemical messages between nerve cells). In particular, this medication seems to stimulate the release of the neurotransmitter called serotonin, and it also increases the effectiveness of another neurotransmitter, noradrenaline. Thus the medication reduces pain conduction by the nerves. Tramadol hydrochlorothide has a powerful effect on fairly severe pain, and its risk of addiction, as previously noted, is markedly less than those of the other narcotic analgesics we have mentioned.

Steroids

Great controversy also surrounds the use of steroids in treating patients with low back pain. While most physicians currently treating back pain syndromes would agree that strategic injections of local steroids will effectively reduce sciatica (back pain that radiates down the leg), opinions vary on the use of steroids in treating low back pain without sciatica.

The previously mentioned 1994 study by the U.S. Department of Health and Human Services suggests that these medications are ineffective for low back pain, even when there is sciatica. Yet other studies have produced other findings. The literature is certainly not conclusive on this issue.

In our practice, we do not use oral steroids for nonradiating acute low back pain. But if a patient has a documented radiculopathy (pinched nerve) with distinct leg symptoms, we feel that a short course of oral steroids will frequently help to reduce pain and to get the person moving again, the importance of which is not disputed.

Muscle Relaxants

Many doctors use muscle relaxants in the management of low back pain. The decision to administer a muscle relaxant is based on the belief that reducing muscle spasm—involuntary contraction of the muscle—will decrease the pain. Unfortunately, research on this subject does not clearly justify the use of these substances.

During muscle spasm, the pressure inside the muscle rises, reducing the amount of blood flowing through the region. Because the blood is not carrying them away, waste products accumulate in the muscle cells and irritate nerve endings.

As the spasm resolves, the pain usually lessens. However, it is not clear whether the medications used as muscle relaxants act directly on the target organ, that is, the spasming muscles. What we do know with certainty is that all of these medications cause drowsiness, which in itself might reduce the muscle spasm. In fact, some physicians have suggested that the effectiveness of this medication is due to its ability to induce sleep, considering that insomnia is often a major problem for people suffering from acute low back pain.

At this time, the action of muscle relaxants is not understood, and no direct effect on muscle tissue has ever been documented. One possibility is that some types of muscle relaxants may interfere with various reflex pathways involved in muscle contraction, thus reducing pain. Further research is needed in this area.

The 1994 government study found that muscle relaxants were somewhat effective in the treatment of acute low back pain but no more so than nonsteroidal medications. Moreover, the study could find no justification for using nonsteroidal drugs and muscle relaxants in combination. The panel reported excessive drowsiness from muscle relaxants in up to 30 percent of the patients studied.

Muscle relaxants can be fairly toxic, especially to the liver. Furthermore, it is possible that the muscle spasm is a part of the healing process. Clearly, additional investigation is required before we can conclude whether these agents may be of use in the treatment of back pain.

Among the many muscle relaxants on the market, cyclobenzaprine (brand name Flexeril) may be the most frequently prescribed. Other common choices include carisoprodol (Soma), chlorzoxazone (Paraflex or Parafon Forte), orphenadrine citrate (Norflex), metaxalone (Skelaxin), methocarbamol (Robaxin), and diazepam (Valium).

Most clinicians agree that the use of these medications is best limited to cases of fairly acute low back pain. On the other hand, we have found that cyclobenzaprine (Flexeril) has sometimes been helpful for patients with chronic low back pain. In fact, we have encountered great resistance from patients when we suggested discontinuing this medication. Yet comparative studies have not shown cyclobenzaprine to be superior to the other drugs.

The most obvious side effect of these medications is drowsiness, a problem that often leads to the termination of this therapy. Blurred vision, headaches, and dizziness are also quite common. Orphenadrine may have the potential to cause cardiac arrhythmia (irregular heartbeats), even in individuals with no known cardiac disease, as well as mental confusion in elderly patients.

Patients with chronic low back pain are susceptible to depression and drug dependency. This fact probably makes diazepam a poor choice as a muscle relaxant because it tends to be both depressive and addictive. There has also been some suggestion that use of carisoprodol tends to lead to addiction, although we have not yet seen substantial proof of this.

Sleeping Medications

People with severe low back pain often have trouble sleeping. We believe that sleep is a part of the healing process and always ask our patients about their sleeping patterns, which may be interrupted by pain, changes in daily activities, medications, and other factors, including depression.

We feel that the short-term use of oral sleeping medications can be valuable. Over-the-counter drugs such as diphenhydramine HCI (Benadryl) may help you to sleep, as may some of the antidepressant medications that we discuss in the last section of this chapter. When choosing a sleeping pill, be sure to first talk to your doctor about the various types, the appropriate dosage, and the length of time you will take the drug. Keep in mind that prolonged use of over-the-counter medications can be dangerous. Just because you don't need a prescription for a certain drug doesn't mean that it's safe for you.

In our practice, we have had wonderful results with zolpidem tartrate (Ambien), an oral sleeping agent that is relatively new to the market. Available in five- and ten-milligram doses, it appears to be quite effective for inducing sleep. This prescribed medication seems to help reset the patient's sleep cycle, quicken the onset of sleep, and make sleep last longer. Despite our extensive use of this therapy, we have observed no negative side effects, and we have had a great many thankful patients.

You have probably read or heard about melatonin, a substance you can buy in health food stores. This is a hormone that some people take to induce sleep. Melatonin is naturally produced in the human body by the pineal gland, and it appears to be involved in modulating various bodily functions, including reproduction. Changes in the release of this substance may regulate not only development during puberty but also ovulation in women. In addition, abnormal release of melatonin may play a role in such disorders as anorexia nervosa and depression.

Melatonin, which is available in tablet and other forms, has been recommended as a "natural" sleep-inducing medication. But until more research is done, we advise caution. If you're interested in using melatonin, discuss the possibility with your physician before trying it.

Keep in mind that the body's hormonal systems are extremely complex and indiscriminate use of sleep-inducing chemicals can cause changes in endocrine (glandular) function. The physical problems that result from the abuse of steroids offer a good example of this.

Colchicine

An extract of the crocus plant, colchicine has been used to treat arthritic conditions since the sixth century. According to some accounts, Benjamin Franklin, who suffered from gout, brought an early form of this medication to the United States.

While we feel that colchicine is useful in treating attacks of gouty arthritis, we have not found it to be helpful for the garden-variety low back condition, which typically responds more favorably to NSAIDs. Some clinicians still use this medication for arthritic conditions other than gout, but recent studies have found it ineffective for the treatment of acute low back pain.

Antidepressants

Doctors use antidepressant medications in the management of many conditions that involve chronic pain, including those affecting the low back. These medications can actually work indirectly as pain relievers (analgesics) because of their direct effect on depressive states. As a depressed person's mood is elevated, this person tends to find his or her pain less troublesome.

Depression is a common and predictable consequence of many chronic conditions. Severe pain alone can drive individuals to despair. Other aspects of chronically painful conditions also contribute to emotional misery. For example, people with chronic pain often have difficulty sleeping at night, and this is a significant risk factor for depression.

A person with chronic pain may be unable to work, which robs him or her of a source of self-esteem. The person may also feel alienated from loved ones, who may not understand the medical condition, may fail to empathize, and may think, "He/she looks just fine to me!" In addition, enjoyable recreational pursuits may become a thing of the past for someone suffering from chronic back pain. The person finds that he or she is no longer able to engage in favorite sports and hobbies, play with the children, or perform everyday chores such as housecleaning, driving, and shopping. Added to this unfortunate collection of experiences are the financial disasters that often befall patients with chronic low back syndromes. Needless to say, if you can't work, your income drops.

Doctors frequently find that the depression resulting from a chronically painful condition is worse than the original malady. Hence any physician treating ailments that cause persistent pain must be knowledgeable about which antidepressants are available and how best to use them.

The first generation of medications that proved effective for depression were the tricyclic antidepressants, named for their three-ringed molecular structure. Examples of these include amitriptyline, imipramine, nortriptyline, and desipramine.

Early studies suggested that these antidepressants had a direct analgesic effect in many painful conditions. Yet the pain relief was often marginal, and major side effects typically led to dosage reduction or discontinuation. Some of the problems were extreme light-headedness, weight gain, drowsiness, blurred vision, dry mouth, and, particularly in men, difficulty urinating. Interactions with other medications also made these antidepressants less than ideal.

The past decade has seen a virtual revolution in antidepressant therapy. Among the many new antidepressants on the scene are venlafaxine (Effexor), fluoxetine (Prozac), bupropion (Wellbutrin), sertraline (Zoloft), nefazodone (Serzone), and paroxetine (Paxil).

While these medications also have some side effects, they truly represent a quantum leap in the treatment of depression, regardless of the cause. Some of these antidepressants appear to make the transfer of pain impulses less efficient. For example, venlafaxine, which became available quite recently, appears to affect both of the body's major mechanisms for conveying pain. When you are in severe pain, a medication that makes your pain conveyors less efficient is a good thing!

Further research on these antidepressants is clearly necessary. We anticipate that the results of future studies will lead to a larger role for these medications in the successful management of both painful back conditions and associated depressive symptoms.

7

Non-Pharmacologic Treatments

It's a good idea to try everything that might improve your back problem. Why not supplement your medical treatment, exercise program, and medications with other therapies? You have an abundance of choices.

One of our patients, referred to us from a regional spine center, was a man in his early seventies who was suffering from wear-and-tear changes of the lower spine. Many local physicians had told him that he would just have to live with his pain, but he refused to believe this. At the spine center, he underwent an extensive and elaborate diagnostic evaluation. This included x-rays, a bone scan, an MRI, a CT scan, and nerve and muscle studies. After going through all these tests, he was again told, "Nothing can be done. You will just have to live with this."

He was understandably disappointed and annoyed about going through all this for nothing. So he came to us in the hope that we had the answers. We explained that we would do what we could for him, but that we could make no promises after so many other qualified specialists had investigated his problem and come up empty-handed.

We ultimately found that he did indeed have degenerative joint changes of the spine but that he also had joint inflammation and facet syndrome. We treated him with a trigger block and a facet block (injections to relieve tightness), and he began an exercise program to strengthen his low back.

We are happy to report that today this patient is feeling much better and can pursue many more activities. Specifically, he can participate in—and enjoy—such social activities as golfing with friends and going to the shopping mall with his wife. These may sound like trivial improvements, but this man was delighted that he could do these things again.

Medication Treatments

Some medications are injected directly into painful areas. We are including these treatments in this chapter (rather than in the chapter on medications) because the physician must carefully administer the drug—the patient cannot simply take a pill, as with other medications.

Trigger Point Injections

Trigger points are areas of muscle contraction, or spasm, that frequently develop after muscular injury. A physician can actually feel a small area of contracted muscle tissue embedded in the surrounding normal muscle tissue.

Trigger points are very tender even when the muscle is at rest. The increased tension in the trigger point accelerates the metabolism of the muscle cells while decreasing the blood flow, making it more difficult for the body to restore important raw materials to the muscle and to wash away waste products. As a result, it is thought that these substances accumulate, irritating nerve fibers and resulting in pain.

Painful trigger points frequently radiate to other areas that may be fairly remote from the original area of muscle spasm. In the lumbar area, trigger points can be found in many places, including the paraspinal muscles and the gluteal muscles (buttocks). Pain in these points can radiate down the leg, simulating sciatica.

If a doctor injects a local anesthetic directly into a trigger point, the trigger point tends to relax. As the muscle spasm ceases, normal blood flow returns to the area. Local anesthetics such as marcaine, procaine, and novocaine are commonly used for trigger point injections. Some physicians favor mixing steroids with the local anesthetic, although others do not feel that this is helpful. After the injection, the doctor may spray the area with a cooling substance and stretch it manually.

We frequently perform this technique in our spine center, with excellent results. Trigger point injections can also be quite useful in the treatment of painful neck muscles.

Epidural Steroid Injections

If tests show that someone with back and leg pain has a pinched nerve, the doctor may administer an epidural steroid injection. This treatment is helpful only for patients with documented nerve root compression and associated leg pain. Steroids are used in this procedure because they can actually reduce inflammation in the involved nerve root—and with this action, the pain is reduced as well. The results may be experienced for weeks or even months, which allows the patient to exercise and recondition his or her back in the hopes of preventing future inflammation.

In this procedure, a locally acting steroid is injected at the site of the pinched nerve. This typically reduces the leg pain but does not do much for the low back pain. Complications are rare but can include local infection or bleeding, post-lumbar puncture headache, and even meningitis.

In the case of the headache, which is similar to the headache many women have after being given an epidural during childbirth, the patient experiences intense headache when sitting upright. The condition is easily treated by infiltrating the area of the needle puncture with a small amount of the patient's own blood; this leads to a local inflammatory reaction, sealing a leak in the spinal membrane.

The scientific basis for epidural steroid injections is somewhat tenuous, and this type of therapy is clearly not for everyone. In particular, this procedure would be a poor choice for someone with a serious neurologic problem such as evident leg weakness, unless he or she should not undergo surgery for some reason, perhaps a heart condition. People with mild sciatica might have better results with therapies other than the epidural injections, although someone with severe sciatica should probably receive this type of injection as soon as a doctor has discovered an anatomic basis for the pain.

In our clinic, we administer the injection three times to an appropriate candidate, usually over a five- to seven-day interval. This allows time to monitor the clinical response to each injection. Salt and fluid retention as well as elevated blood sugar levels may occur, but with appropriate management these side effects can be readily addressed.

Facet Joint Injections

The facet joints (the smaller joints between adjacent vertebrae) can generate severe low back pain. Because these joints are very small, they are difficult to localize blindly with a needle. The doctor therefore needs to employ some kind of imaging technique in order to locate the proper place for the injection.

In our clinic, we perform this type of injection using a modified x-ray technique or a CT scan. The needle doesn't have to go directly in the joint; in fact, the injection is probably more effective if the needle is placed very near to the joint. Usually the injection is a "cocktail" of a steroid and a local anesthetic.

Many practitioners suggest that two adjacent facet joints be blocked (receive injections) at the same time, because a facet joint typically receives pain messages from two different spinal nerves. This injection is for short-term reduction of inflammation in the joint.

In recent years, medical experts have criticized facet blocks as ineffective for the long-term treatment of low back pain. It's true that studies on the long-range results of this therapy have not clearly demonstrated its validity. But we feel that this approach to evaluating facet blocks misses the point.

If a procedure reduces the number of days a person stays in bed and allows him or her to get started on an exercise program early in the course of treatment, this procedure has merit. We feel that the patient's suffering and decreased productivity should receive major consideration from a doctor who is selecting appropriate therapies. While doctors who rigidly go by the book might take issue with our approach, most patients would applaud it. The following story illustrates this.

A thirty-eight-year-old cardiologist came to our clinic as soon as he began to have acute low back pain. He had been forced to cancel all his patients' appointments that day because his pain was so severe. He said that he had felt "fine" the day before, but on the day he saw us, he had awakened with severe pain to the right of his lower lumbar spine; the pain radiated into the buttock and back of the thigh but not below the knee.

He had not experienced any weakness or numbness; his pain didn't worsen on coughing or sneezing; and he had no symptoms on the left side. During the physical examination, we found some muscle spasm in the right side of the lower lumbar region, and he had trouble with the straight-leg-raising test. He had exquisite tenderness over the lowest part of the lumbar spine and the highest part of the sacrum. An x-ray showed that bony lumbar anatomy was normal.

We immediately administered a facet block, and he responded quite well. He felt some local pain after the injection but reported an approximately 90 percent reduction in the pain that had brought him to see us. We instructed him on how to perform some stretching exercises at home, which he agreed to do. The next day, this man was able to resume his physically demanding work in the cardiac lab.

Facet Rhizotomy

If repeated facet blocks successfully alleviate the patient's pain, though only temporarily despite implementation of a relevant exercise program, the nerves sending pain messages from the facet joint can be destroyed (facet rhizotomy) by various means. In this therapy, a needle probe is placed near the nerves supplying the facet joint, and energy is then applied to the area in the form of radio-frequency waves or heat. Less frequently, irritating substances are injected in a similar manner to destroy the nerve fibers. While this outpatient treatment can lead to very dramatic results, patient selection is crucial and is best left in the hands of experienced back care specialists.

Non-Medication Treatments

Some people are averse to taking medications, including aspirin or acetaminophen. And even if you don't balk at taking the occasional aspirin, you would probably like to know whether there are any non-medication actions you can take to lessen your back pain. In fact, there are many, including several you may never have considered.

Shoe Lifts and Insoles

There's a simple way to help your low back that rarely occurs to people. You can get fitted with a shoe lift or an insole that evens out the length of your legs.

Solid evidence shows that dissimilar leg length can lead to chronic low back pain. If your legs differ in length by less than two centimeters, these devices are not likely to be helpful. But if you have a larger discrepancy, you may find that a lift for your shorter leg makes a noticeable difference in your back.

These devices are very inexpensive and often worth a try. Talk to your doctor or podiatrist about them.

Postural Training

Poor posture is unquestionably a risk factor for low back pain and presumably makes the pain of an already injured back even worse. Without realizing it, you may sit or stand in a way that significantly increases the pressure on your low back.

You can break the habits of poor posture just as you can break other unhealthy habits, but what really helps is to strengthen the muscles that hold your body upright. Chapter 5 offers valuable exercises to help condition these muscles; follow the exercise plan presented there to strengthen your back and improve your posture.

Biofeedback

This is a fairly labor-intensive type of training that is occasionally helpful for people with severe chronic low back pain. Mastery of biofeedback is demanding, not only for the patient but also for the therapist.

Biofeedback is a technique through which a person develops some mental control over involuntary processes in the body, thus decreasing his or her own pain. Various auditory and visual signals guide the patient's responses as he or she develops this ability. The therapy has its supporters, although studies have not clearly documented it as an effective treatment for back pain.

Relaxation therapy and hypnosis also have supporters. Although we have found these types of therapies to be fairly ineffective in alleviating all of a patient's pain, they can be helpful in a limited way. Such therapies may also help with muscle relaxation.

Bed Rest

In the past, the standard treatment for back pain was to order the patient to stay in bed for days. This is no longer true. Instead, most back pain experts today feel that the role of bed rest has been greatly overstressed in the management of back pain conditions.

The current consensus is that two to three days of bed rest are the *maximum* amount of time for cessation of normal activity. If you are inactive for longer than this period, your nerves and muscles begin to degenerate, your heart and lungs lose fitness, and your bones become more porous and fragile. And those are just the physical effects. Staying in bed for days is demoralizing for even the cheeriest types, and if you're not naturally optimistic, you may start to despair of ever being active and pain-free again. An early resumption of normal activities is absolutely essential to a quick, complete recovery.

Exercise

Instead of resting in bed, you need to become active again. In fact, you probably need to become more active than you were before your back pain began.

The reason is that, like a majority of the patients with back pain syndromes, you likely have weak back muscles. The goal of exercise is not to reduce pain per se, but by improving muscular function, strength, flexibility, and endurance, you may eliminate one of the main reasons your back hurts. In addition, by continuing to exercise, you can avoid getting caught in the cycle of chronic disuse atrophy, in which you rest because your back hurts, your back muscles become even weaker from the inactivity, and your back hurts even more.

The benefits of exercise are numerous: Exercise decreases the physical stress on various structures in your spine, raises your general fitness level, reduces your psychological stress, decreases your anxiety over having chronic back pain, improves your posture, and enhances your mobility. These positive changes motivate you to continue exercising, which in turn leads to continued improvement in all of these physical and emotional aspects of your health. Ultimately, these changes lead to a reduction in your pain and your perception of pain.

A study published in the *Journal of Occupational Medicine* explored the relationship between general physical fitness and low back pain. The study found that among a large number of firefighters, those with high physical fitness had very few back injuries, while those with low physical fitness had a significantly higher rate of injury. Thus physical fitness plays a role not only in recovery from injuries but in preventing them.

Over the last few decades, many physicians have prescribed what was the standard treatment for back pain: rest, passive therapies, medicines, and stretching—and, if all of these failed, treatment at a pain clinic. We now know that the best way to treat nonmalignant, nonstructural causes of back pain is with aggressive therapy and exercises to strengthen weak muscles. If you have low back pain, exercise is not just a good idea; it is absolutely essential to overcoming your condition.

Chiropractic

This system of therapy, in which skeletal structures are manipulated with the aim of restoring normal nerve function, is one of the most controversial areas in modern medicine. Chiropractic is highly revered by many patients and just as reviled by many traditional medical doctors. In many medical schools, if instructors mention chiropractic at all, they present it in a negative light. Students hear that chiropractic causes strokes and that chiropractors make inappropriate adjustments and cause delays in the initiation of correct therapies for diseases that require emergency medical care. Even among chiropractors, there is enormous difference of opinion with regard to most aspects of chiropractic treatment.

Despite all this dissension, the profession thrives in terms of the number of people who receive chiropractic treatment each year. Furthermore, in recent years, we have seen a significant improvement in the relations between the mainstream medical establishment and the chiropractic profession. Chiropractic has clearly been validated as a treatment for many musculoskeletal conditions in respected medical journals such as the *British Medical Journal,* in reports from the private sector by such institutions as the Rand Corporation, and, more recently, by governmental agencies including the U.S. Department of Health and Human Services. Ultimately, numerous medical authorities have concluded that, whatever it is chiropractors are doing, their treatments can bring significant improvement to certain musculoskeletal conditions. In our practice, we frequently refer patients for chiropractic care and have been very pleased with the outcomes we have seen.

The components of chiropractic treatment and how they work are subjects that are poorly understood. While chiropractors do various types of therapy, including massage, ultrasound, heat, and exercise instruction, their primary maneuvers are mobilization and manipulation.

A chiropractor mobilizes a joint by moving it to the point where motion is restricted by the joint itself or by its supporting tissues (ligaments and muscles). Manipulation takes that movement slightly beyond this normal range of motion. In a single act of manipulation, called an adjustment, the chiropractor usually moves or bears down on an area of the patient's body.

Chiropractors frequently invoke the concept of *subluxation* as the basis for their treatments. A subluxation is an improper alignment of the joint surfaces. The theory is that this partial dislocation can lead to pain, muscle spasm, and stiffness, all of which causes the person with the condition to avoid activity. The manipulative adjustments of chiropractic are intended to restore proper alignment of the joint surfaces and reduce the pain-generating process.

To illustrate the concept of subluxation, imagine grasping one of your fingers with the opposite hand and rotating the finger slightly (we do not recommend actually doing this). At some point, the rotatory force would move your finger's joints beyond their normal range of motion. This would produce pain, and the pain would increase with the degree of rotational force you apply.

The failure of medical science to explain the efficacy of chiropractic treatment is not without precedent. Established medicine often endorses remedies and dispenses advice that work for reasons no one yet understands, and it is certainly not uncommon for two MDs to give virtually opposite pieces of advice to the same patient about a particular condition. This situation underscores the absolute necessity of educating yourself about your own condition as well as about the available treatments.

We feel that the chiropractic profession has been greatly harmed by the public activities of some chiropractors. For example, certain chiropractors promise to remedy middle ear infections, narrowed arteries and heart disease, and many other conditions that can have serious consequences if they don't receive appropriate and timely treatment. Through radio and television commercials, these chiropractic sirens barrage the public with their fallacious claims, while their more knowledgeable, ethical, and serious colleagues watch this behavior, aghast and embarrassed. Unfortunately, some medical doctors have reacted to the vocal chiropractors' falsehoods by dismissing the entire profession. This is similar to condemning all medical doctors because some of them are incompetent or unethical. We believe most doctors are good at what they do and that most chiropractors are also competent.

When we feel that a patient would benefit from some type of manual therapy, we do not hesitate to refer him or her to one of the many local chiropractors with whom we have a working relationship. Because chiropractors cannot prescribe medication, the combination of a medical doctor and a chiropractor can provide a patient with well-rounded and effective treatment. Our patients seem to benefit just from knowing that we are open to this as a therapy option. And if one or two chiropractic treatments do not resolve a patient's pain, we often recommend having additional sessions or going to see a different chiropractor.

Finally, we should note that chiropractic adjustments are occasionally made under anesthesia. Scar tissue can form in tendons, muscles, and joint capsules. When this happens, a forceful adjustment to restore range of motion to the area can be too painful for a conscious patient. This type of therapy, called manipulation under anesthesia, has its supporters, who argue convincingly for its value.

To our knowledge, no scientific studies have documented the efficacy of this treatment. However, orthopedic surgeons frequently perform manipulation under general anesthesia as part of the treatment of so-called frozen shoulder syndrome. This is a problem that often complicates painful shoulder conditions, whether they arose from local trauma, heart attack, or even a pinched nerve in the neck. Generally, manipulation of the shoulder under anesthesia restores normal, pain-free motion to the joint.

Acupuncture

In this ancient Chinese treatment, the practitioner inserts needles at certain points on the patient's body with the goal of curing ailments or alleviating pain. Although modern scientists don't know precisely how it works, acupuncture may lead to the release of endorphins and enkephalins, which are painkilling proteins in the brain. These biochemicals are our own personal opiates, and our bodies release them when we have pain. They are also released during exercise and can produce a temporary euphoria that is often referred to as a "runner's high."

Eastern medicine has long used acupuncture to relieve and prevent pain sensations. It has sometimes been used during surgery to block pain. Acupuncture is widely available through the United States, the UK, and Canada, and your family doctor should be able to refer you to a competent practitioner.

Traction

Traction is essentially the use of weights and harnesses to stretch the injured portion of the spine. In the remote past, this was a standard inpatient treatment for back pain. Hospitalized patients were made to stay in uncomfortable positions for seemingly endless periods of time. The cure was truly worse than the disease.

Prolonged use of this therapy leads to loss of muscle tissue, loss of minerals from bones, blood clots in the legs, and all the other complications of prolonged bed rest. Some variations of traction therapy may even raise the risks of elevated blood pressure and increased pressure inside the eye.

These days, this type of therapy is used on an outpatient basis. A harness is attached to the pelvis, and a cord is attached to the harness; the cord goes over a pulley with various amount of weights attached to the other end. The goal is theoretically to reduce the pressure on the painful joints, nerve roots, and muscles, or possibly to reduce the pressure inside the intervertebral disc or discs.

The U.S. Department of Health and Human Services recently suggested that traction is not helpful in the treatment of acute low back pain. Our belief is that it can be useful for patients who definitely have nerve root compression (a pinched nerve) and for whom other treatments, such as epidural steroid injections, have failed. We do not recommend this therapy for patients who don't have clearly documented radiculopathy.

Orthotic Devices (Corsets and Braces)

Like most treatments of low back pain, the use of braces and corsets is a hotbed of controversy. Even people who are considered experts in the field of treating low back problems have differing opinions on this therapy. A recent government study has suggested that lumbar corsets have no proven benefit for people suffering from acute low back problems, though it also indicated that wearing these devices may have some value as a preventive measure.

These back supports come in many shapes and styles—from the firm leather weight lifter's belt to the wide, elasticized supporter you may have seen at home supply centers or worn by some hospital employees.

The rationale for use of orthotic devices is that they reduce the motion of the lumbar spine, leading to diminished irritation. If worn tightly, a lumbar corset can also increase the pressure in the abdomen, which may indirectly relieve the compression in the low back area.

We have not found these devices to be helpful for our patients, whether their back pain is acute or chronic. Yet we agree with the study that suggested orthotics may help to prevent low back injuries in people doing heavy lifting. In our experience, however, these devices are rarely used appropriately. So, if heavy lifting is part of your job or an unavoidable activity for some other reason, talk to your doctor about using a lumbar corset, and ask him or her to instruct you on how to use it correctly.

Ultrasound

Using high-frequency vibrations, this painless procedure can stimulate blood flow and reduce inflammation in affected areas. Ultrasound can reach tissues up to two inches below the skin's surface, giving it the advantage of deeper penetration than most other therapies. The energy applied by the ultrasonic instrument may have an effect similar to that of heat therapy.

While some patients feel that ultrasound lessens their low back pain, medical research has not clearly supported this therapy's usefulness. Occasionally, ultrasound therapy is used to transmit a local steroid ointment, such as prednisolone, to help reduce inflammation. There is also no clear documentation of this therapy's worth.

Cryotherapy

Another therapy that has not been proven to be effective but has many patient advocates is cryotherapy, which is simply the application of cold to painful areas. Cryotherapy is typically used for acute conditions in which inflammation is fairly intense. The penetrating cold appears to narrow the blood vessels, which would tend to reduce swelling (or edema, as doctors call it) as well as muscle spasm. The low temperature can also lessen the efficiency of the nerves in transmitting impulses, reducing the sensation of pain.

In this therapy, ice packs are usually applied to the painful area. Cryotherapy can also be performed with ice massage (moving ice gently over the skin) and even with an ethyl chloride spray (a surface anesthetic). Usually, after a few minutes, the feeling of cold gives way to a sensation of heat or burning and, ultimately, to numbness.

Many people with chronic low back pain feel that ice has helped them, while many others feel that heat works better. Still others feel better from alternating the two types of therapy. The perceived benefits may simply be related to a person's strong desire to take action—to do *something* for his or her condition.

The best approach, therefore, may be to experiment. First see whether you can stand having an ice pack on your low back; if you can, see whether applying it for twenty minutes eases your pain. Another time, you may want to try applying heat, so that you can compare your responses to the two treatments. If you wish to try alternating the two, we recommend ice for twenty minutes, nothing for one hour, heat for twenty to forty minutes, and nothing for one hour. You can then repeat this cycle.

Heat

The application of heat is a time-honored treatment for low back pain. It is thought to expand blood vessels in the area, allowing the blood to carry away metabolic irritants and bring nutrients to the healing tissue. Heat tends to make the soft tissues more flexible and to reduce the pain.

Moist heat (applied through wettable heating pads, hot showers, or whirlpool baths) tends to be more effective than dry heat (using a heating pad that can't be moistened). An application generally lasts no longer than twenty to forty minutes.

Heat therapy works better for chronic pain than it does for acute pain from an injury. Unfortunately, the applied heat does not penetrate beyond the layer of fat beneath the skin.

An alternative to this superficial type of heat delivery is diathermy. This therapy uses electromagnetic currents in the microwave range to penetrate to the underlying tissues. In many cases, this directed heat therapy is more helpful than warming rubs, lotions, or creams, or heating pads.

Massage

In treating someone with low back pain, a massage therapist applies pressure to the muscles of the low back area. This is also called manual therapy because the practitioner uses his or her hands to manipulate and adjust the patient's spine.

The goals of massage therapy are to promote blood flow, to decrease muscle spasm and pain, and to promote a general sense of well-being. As we have mentioned elsewhere, muscle spasm can restrict blood flow, allowing irritating substances to accumulate in the muscles and stimulate nerve endings, which leads to the perception of pain.

No study has indicated that massage therapy alone can alter the long-term outcome of any back pain syndrome. Massage is frequently combined with other therapeutic techniques, however, and this strategy can be quite effective in providing pain relief, perhaps particularly in cases of exacerbated chronic back pain.

Electrical Treatments

In the recent past, some practitioners have used electrical treatments to stimulate areas of pain and, theoretically, to reduce the pain. The results of this type of treatment have been mixed, and its efficacy remains in question.

Transcutaneous Electrical Nerve Stimulations (TENS)

The so-called TENS unit is a small, battery-operated device that you can wear or with which you can be treated on an outpatient basis at a clinic. A TENS unit provides the low back with continuous electrical impulses that can vary in frequency and wave pattern and that seem to relieve pain. (*Transcutaneous*, if you're wondering, simply means passing through the skin.)

There are various explanations for how this treatment lessens pain, including the release of endorphins (the same natural painkillers released during acupuncture) and the overstimulation of nerve endings. The theory on overstimulation is the following: Basically, all pain messages have to be relayed to the brain. If the stimulator produces intense sensations of numbness, this message may get to the brain first and block the additional pain messages from getting through. An applicable analogy is the method of hitting your thumb with a hammer to get rid of a headache.

A recent government study has suggested that this treatment is ineffective for acute low back pain. This is a very safe type of therapy, however, and if your pain isn't severe, you may want to try it, though certainly not as your sole form of therapy. One caveat: If you have a cardiac pacemaker, you should not receive transcutaneous electrical nerve stimulations.

Iontophoresis

In contrast to the alternating type of current used with the TENS unit, iontophoresis involves applying a direct electric current to the area of pain. This is typically used with a variety of medications, including not only corticosteroids but local anesthetics and even adrenaline.

As with most treatments, this therapy has its supporters, but our patients have not had favorable results. Clearly, it is insufficient as the only treatment for your problem, since it deals with relieving pain but does nothing to locate the cause, remedy any abnormal conditions, or strengthen weak muscles.

8

When Surgery Is Necessary

Although surgery is rarely either the patient's or the physician's first choice, it is still sometimes the best option. Surgery is expensive, and the recuperation period can be painful and lengthy. According to Metropolitan Life Insurance Company's 1995 analysis of hundreds of thousands of medical claims in the United States, the average hospital and physician fees for back surgery were about $14,000 in 1993, with wide variations among states.

If you suffer from chronic back pain, you may be confused about whether surgery can help you. Or perhaps you take an extreme view, believing either that it will make you worse or that it will cure you completely. In our experience, opinions on back surgery are polarized at one end or the other. Among our patients, those who wish to discuss this option begin either by saying, "I know someone who had surgery and couldn't walk afterwards," or by saying, "I have a friend who suffered for years with back pain. He had surgery, and since that time he's been doing great."

The truth about surgery is that most of the time it provides reasonable benefits to patients who have been appropriately selected. It is seldom either a miracle cure or a complete failure. We have two basic guidelines for our patients who clearly have an abnormal change in structure because of injury or disease. We recommend surgery in the following cases:

1. If an extremity shows progressive weakness that is probably caused by an identified problem in the back (such as a ruptured disc).
2. If there is intractable pain.

These indicators are not absolute, and there are certainly many factors to consider when deciding on surgery. Yet these are reasonable standards that have helped us decide whether to advise surgery, particularly in difficult cases. Of course, we refer a potential candidate for surgery to a neurosurgeon who will make an independent evaluation of whether surgery could help this patient's back.

Spine surgery performed for the sole purpose of relieving pain is notoriously ineffective, as has been documented by the medical literature on this subject. We do not recommend surgery if there is no obvious anatomic cause for the pain syndrome, and we certainly don't recommend that you go "under the knife" just so your doctor can take a look and see what's wrong.

Before you read about the various surgeries, it is important for you to know that the surgical options have come a long way since the days when we started to practice medicine. (And we are both young men—one in his thirties, the other in his forties.) Years ago, our patients who had back surgery would often remain in bed for weeks afterward and would then endure a very slow healing process. Today, except for those with the most extreme conditions, patients are encouraged to be active within days or even hours of undergoing surgery, and a lengthy hospital stay is seldom necessary.

As you try to understand the various surgeries, remember the analogy of the jelly doughnut. If the doughnut moves backwards or sideways, as in a bulging disc, the surgeon often simply needs to make room for the nerve or spinal cord to exit through an opening, thereby relieving pressure from the compressed nerve or spinal cord. On the other hand, if the nucleus pulposus (the central gooey part of the disc) ruptures or explodes through the fibrous outer part, like the jelly bursting through when you squeeze the doughnut, this often creates additional problems, and a more complicated surgical intervention may be necessary.

Surgical Procedures

Let's assume that your neurologist or other specialist has taken a thorough medical history, performed a physical examination, and ordered diagnostic tests. Assume further that the test results confirmed the initial diagnosis. The physician has found the location of your sciatica or nerve root problem, and you are ready for surgery. Which procedure will you have?

The choice will be based on your body size and general physical condition, as well as various aspects of your problem that were observed by the doctor or discovered through clinical testing. These may include the type of disc displacement, the degree of joint inflammation or bone spur formation, and the specific location of calcium deposits.

Disc Removal

If an intervertebral disc is bulging or ruptured, your surgeon may choose to do the classic disc removal operation, which is a very frequently performed procedure. You will be positioned flat on your stomach so that the surgeon can make an incision at the base of your spine.

To reach the disc, your surgeon will actually remove some of the vertebral bone. He or she will then remove some of the disc material, allowing the trapped nerve roots to exit more freely. The scar from this procedure is usually a few inches long.

Microdiscectomy

For a bulging or ruptured disc, your surgeon may consider a procedure that is similar to the classic disc removal but is done using a microscope for magnification. This allows the surgeon to make a much smaller incision, with far less tissue irritation and considerably less destruction of bone.

This microsurgery can sometimes be performed on an outpatient basis, and recovery tends to be quite rapid. The scar will be small, anywhere from half an inch to one-and-a-half inches in length.

Bone Removal

In either the classic disc removal or the microdiscectomy, the surgeon will need to remove a portion of bone to reach the disc material. This can be done in a number of ways, including a laminotomy, which is basically the removal of part of the lamina, a section of the vertebral bone. Removing this creates an opening through which the surgeon can manipulate disc material and even move nerve roots out of the way.

Sometimes the surgeon needs to remove additional bone to make more room. In this situation, bone spurs or narrowing of the spinal canal (spinal stenosis) may be cramping the spinal cord or nerve roots. If there is a great deal of bony overgrowth, the surgeon may choose to remove the entire lamina, which is called a laminectomy. If this has to be done over more than one or two segments, it often leads to an unstable spine. (It would only be done if there were problems at multiple spine levels.)

Spinal Fusion

If the surgeon decides to do a laminectomy on more than one vertebra, he may consider doing a fusion, which is basically what you would suppose it to be—a joining together of the vertebrae. The surgeon uses some special material to fuse the spine, and although mobility is lost at that joint, the overall stability of the spine remains intact.

In the past, bone was taken from the patient's own pelvic girdle and used in the fusion. Because a surgical procedure was needed to collect this bone, the patient had to undergo two operations and thus ended up with two scars. The bone was crumbled up and placed as a type of epoxy to act as an agent in the fusion.

Many additional sources for bone have since been found, one of which is the bodies of people who have just died. With growing concern over the transmission of hepatitis and AIDS, however, this method has fallen out of favor. Fortunately, scientists recently identified a new and exciting option. This material is not human bone at all but a type of sea coral. Experimental procedures have used sterilized sea coral with positive results, although full approval by the Food and Drug Administration is still pending for spine surgeries. It appears that this may be a viable option in the future.

If the spine becomes too unstable, the fusion procedure may not be enough. Additional fixative devices may be necessary. A surgeon may place metal plates and screws in the remaining bone structures to create stability. This is often part of a second or third spine surgery, particularly after a first or second surgery has failed.

Stabilizing the Spine

We need to address this issue further. When more than one segment of bone is removed or worked on, the spine will be highly susceptible to injury unless some kind of device is used to lend support. Fusion is an option when only small portions of bone have been removed and the danger of instability isn't great. But when the risk of instability rises, the surgeon may have to insert metal devices, bone, or bonelike material into the spine.

Metal Fixative Devices

A great many prosthetic devices are available for stabilizing a spine from which bone has been removed. The most simple of these are, as we said, basically a combination of plates and screws. A surgeon screws this hardware into parts of the spine in order to prevent the bones from moving off their axis or rotating, thus allowing the spine to function safely.

As you may recall from the anatomy chapter, the spinal column houses the spinal cord and the nerve roots, vital structures of the nervous system. If the spine moves in an inappropriate fashion, these nerve structures can be pinched, trapped, or, worst of all, severed. So the surgeon puts these screws and plates in place to keep the spine within its normal range of motion. Unfortunately, over time, with the inevitable motion of a human body, the fixative devices can become loose; furthermore, they can actually cause bone inflammation or irritation as well as formation of additional bone spurs. These possibilities must be considerations in the decision to use plates and screws. If you have this procedure, the area will need to be carefully monitored.

Different surgeons have different preferences for bone fusion devices. If you are having this procedure, ask your surgeon which devices he or she plans to use. These appliances will be in your back for the rest of your life, so you should certainly know their risks as well as their benefits.

Bone Plugs and Other Methods

Sometimes surgeons use bone plugs or bone transplants from cadavers to stabilize the spine. Sea coral, as previously mentioned, may be another possible material.

In addition, there are new medical devices that stimulate bone fusion with electric signals and pulses. In this very experimental procedure, a stimulation device is inserted next to the area on which the surgeon is operating. This accelerates the healing process and causes bone to fuse more readily than it otherwise would. The option to have this procedure has existed for only a short period time, so the long-term effect of the accelerated fusion is unknown. The technique shows promise, however, particularly with regard to shortening the recovery and rehabilitation process.

New Surgical Techniques

Recently some very exciting procedures for back problems have become widely available. In fact, improved techniques are becoming available almost on a weekly or monthly basis. Just as your neurosurgeon should be knowledgeable about these techniques, you should educate yourself about them too, so that you know all your options and can make intelligent choices.

Videoscopic Disc Removal

One important new technique is a disc removal performed with the assistance of a special instrument that allows the surgeon to view the interior of the patient's joints, other structures, and tissues. By watching a television monitor and manipulating this "videoscope," the surgeon can see what he or she is doing without having to open the patient up. Similar to arthroscopic surgery for the knee or shoulder, this disc removal is sometimes called a "Band-Aid surgery" because the operation normally leaves the patient with only a very small puncture mark.

The surgeon usually inserts a suction needle probe (which has a rotating blade and suction capacity) through the puncture site. This probe can enter a disc and actually chew up and remove bulging, distorted, or displaced disc material. Impressively, none of the spinal column bone has to be cut in this procedure, because the surgeon can see the disc material directly with the videoscope and therefore does not need to remove any bone.

This operation is often done on an outpatient basis. When you hear someone say, "Oh, I had back surgery yesterday, and here I am at work today," the person probably had this type of procedure.

Laser Surgery

Currently touted by many as a "cure," laser surgery is the latest technique for treating disc problems in the lumbar spine. While this surgery is performed at some academic centers, it is not widely available to the public. This is primarily because there are problems with the fine control of the laser that's necessary for this procedure, and consequently, there have been some complications. As advancing technology improves the laser, the surgery will become available at more sites.

This technique has considerable promise for helping people who have undergone one or two failed back surgeries and who, as a result of the surgery, have scar tissue. The laser surgery is supposed to produce less scar formation, and this may mean less additional irritation or inflammation of the nerve roots. Also, the laser can actually evaporate prior scar tissue. Keep in mind, however, that this option may not become available for a time and that the long-term results of laser surgery are not fully known.

Disc Transplant

In October 1995, the *Spine Letter,* a magazine dedicated to orthopedic-neurosurgical intervention, published an article titled "Disc Transplantation: A Likely Alternative to Fusion." This cutting-edge study explored the possibility of replacing a removed disc with a disc from a deceased person.

The question that concerned the researchers was whether the transplanted disc would survive. In all but one case, the disc remained adequate, without displacement. The area healed, and there was minimal rejection of the disc material from the body. The material did, however, show some cell degeneration, but the disc retained a great deal of its natural moisture, which is very good. This procedure could become an attractive option for patients who would otherwise need bone fusion after a disc removal.

This leads us to the exciting concept of placing synthetic disc material in the intervertebral regions, particularly when a first or second surgery has failed or when, for physiological reasons, discs continue to degenerate despite medical intervention. Medical research may turn this idea and others into real options in the very near future.

Getting the Most from Surgery

Many patients who come to see us seem to perceive surgery as a cure for their severe chronic low back pain. In reality, surgical procedures can help a fairly small percentage of those with back conditions, and these patients' ailments must meet specific criteria. In particular, we look for the problem of progressive weakness and motor dysfunction in a leg that is caused by a structural change that we have identified through testing. Other possible candidates for surgery may be those who have intractable pain associated with a structural change that is revealed through diagnostic testing.

Before you have any surgical procedure, it's important to understand that surgery may remove the defective disc material, the bulging disc, or even the bone spur that may be causing your pain and localized weakness, but surgery will not address such issues as a deconditioned low back and the resulting soft tissue changes. Talk to your surgeon about what improvement you can hope to gain from a specific surgical procedure and what changes you should not expect. Learn as much as you can about the procedure and how to help yourself recover from it as quickly as possible. People most likely to experience a positive outcome from surgery have the following:

1. Realistic expectations prior to surgery.
2. An understanding of the risks of surgery, which include infection, nerve root irritation or damage, internal bleeding, muscle changes, and increased pain or even scar formation that could cause more problems in the future.
3. Knowledge of what postoperative care and recovery will entail.
4. A thorough understanding of postoperative physical therapy.
5. Education about proper body mechanics.
6. Education about long-term spine care, including how to exercise and condition the back and how to avoid reinjury.

Reluctance to Undergo Surgery

One of Dr. Kandel's patients, who happened to be an adjuster for a workers' compensation company, had been in a motor vehicle collision. Though she wanted to avoid back surgery at first, and continued to work despite severe pain, it was obvious from her MRI and electrodiagnostic studies that she had a pinched nerve in the low back as the result of a ruptured disc.

She finally agreed to have surgery. Within twenty-four hours of the procedure, her terrible back and leg pain had almost completely disappeared. She had mild postsurgical pain, but her operation was clearly a success.

This woman was shocked by how quickly her pain syndrome improved after surgery and by how many activities she was able to resume within a short period. In her work as an adjuster, she had always urged her clients' physicians to take a conservative approach, possibly convincing them to wait longer before intervening surgically than they normally would have. But after seeing her own benefits of less pain and increased function, as well as her shortened disability time and speedy return to work, she was a convert. She told Dr. Kandel, "I guess if you really need surgery, you really need surgery." She has subsequently kept this in mind when dealing with clients who have work-related injuries.

As we have indicated, surgery isn't always so successful and certainly carries risks, but it also has the power to change lives. If your neurologist thinks surgery can help you, don't let fear overwhelm your ability to make a carefully reasoned decision.

When Surgery Is Not Successful

Unfortunately, sometimes surgery does not produce the results the patient had been hoping to experience. It's a good idea to learn about success rates and possible side effects of particular surgeries before making a decision. Whatever you read or hear about a procedure, keep in mind that individuals are different and problems sometimes occur.

Dissatisfaction with the Laminectomy

In recent years, surveys of patients who have undergone lumbar laminectomy, particularly in the treatment of lumbar spinal stenosis, have revealed that a significant proportion are unhappy with the results. (This procedure, as you may recall, involves removing part of the bony spine in the low back in order to widen the spinal canal.) Previously surgeons had believed that patients who underwent this procedure were very pleased with the outcome and would be able to function well.

Two separate studies have indicated this unfavorable opinion of the surgical treatment for lumbar canal stenosis. One of these, published in the November 1994 issue of *Journal of Neurosurgery* and lead by Dr. Tite, produced the following statistics: Only 30 percent of patients felt that their condition was "much improved" from their presurgical condition, 5 percent felt that their condition was "worse" than it had been before the surgery, and 12 percent felt that their condition was "much worse" than it had been beforehand.

Another study, published in a 1995 issue of *Spine* and led by Dr. Jeffrey Katz, revealed that patients who had undergone this same procedure for the same condition felt relatively unsatisfied with the outcome. The subjects for this study, who were referred to Dr. Katz at an academic center, may have had more severe symptoms than patients not requiring academic evaluation. Yet we cannot disregard the fact that so many were not pleased with the results of this surgery.

Second Surgeries

In evaluating back surgery, particularly in the treatment of lumbar spinal stenosis (narrowing of the spinal canal in the low back), it's interesting to compare patients who have undergone one surgery with those who have undergone two. Patients may not heal completely after a first surgery, leaving the question of whether a second surgery is more likely to help or harm them.

A study by Dr. Herno, published in the April 1995 issue of *Spine,* revealed that patients who have already had back surgery have a "highly significant worsening effect of the outcome" compared to patients having their first surgery. Even a well-established diagnosis of spinal stenosis, upon which a physician might base a strong recommendation of surgery, was not an indicator of improvement after a second surgery.

If you have already had surgery for lumbar spinal stenosis and it didn't improve your condition, the results of this study should give you pause. Before deciding to undergo a second procedure, evaluate the pros and cons. Talk to your doctor about the specific reasons that he or she recommends additional surgery in your case.

Surgical Outcomes

Why do so many patients do poorly following surgery? One major reason for a bad surgical outcome is scar formation, which is actually a natural healing process. In the scientific realm, this is called fibrosis, and scarring around the sac that contains the spinal cord and nerve roots is peridural fibrosis.

There is inevitably injury to tissue at the site of a surgical intervention, whether the tissue is deep bone, ligament, tendon, or the covering of the spinal canal (dura mater). This tissue heals by forming a scar. If that scar is too significant, too thick, or too long, or if it forms in the wrong place, it can irritate nerves and cause more problems.

This condition is similar to one with which you may be familiar. Some women who have had hysterectomies have to undergo a second surgery a few years later because adhesions have formed. In other words, tissues that are normally separate have become joined through the scarring process, and this causes all sorts of bowel problems and occasionally bladder problems. The same process can happen in the spinal canal, and therefore, if adhesions can be prevented, the surgery may have a higher chance of success.

The statistics vary depending upon the source, but we can say that back surgery fails for up to 20 percent of patients, and that five years after surgery, a large majority of patients will have additional symptoms requiring ongoing intervention. These statistics are not likely to make anyone feel optimistic, and anything that can be done to reduce the chance of failure or improve the chance of a good outcome is certainly worth exploring.

Reducing Scar Formation

Neurosurgeons have lately discovered that using a certain chemical before closing the surgical wound appears to reduce scarring, as measured by MRI scans. This chemical is a carbohydrate polymer gel, and it is applied directly to the surgical site. A study of this chemical's use in surgery, published in an August 1995 issue of the *Spine Letter,* revealed that if the amount of scarring is reduced, patients have a more positive outcome. In the article, Dr. Dunscur, a neurosurgeon from Cincinnati, was quoted as saying that this "supports the concept that those with more scar have more pain." While this technique is still in its early stages, it shows promise.

What to Keep in Mind After Surgery

Whether or not the outcome of your surgery is considered satisfactory, you'll still need to do certain things during your recovery period to speed your healing process and better your chances of living with little or no pain.

The Early Period

Slow and steady is a good motto for the first few weeks after your surgery. As you might expect, doing too much too fast can actually increase scar formation, cause your wound to open, and create additional problems.

Dr. Kandel had a patient who was himself a medical doctor. After having back surgery, this patient mistakenly assumed he could quickly resume his medical practice. He returned to work, his wound opened, and the bacteria that normally exists on skin entered his body. He ultimately developed not only meningitis but also an abscess in his low back.

This problem required a second surgery and a lengthy course of antibiotics. The antibiotics produced additional systemic side effects, and he felt simply "rotten." When he finally healed, he had a large scar and intractable back pain.

Further surgery was out of the question, because of the significant scar formation, and to this day the patient is on medical disability. He cannot resume a practice that he had trained for and built up over many years and from which he derived immense pleasure. All of this happened because he went back to work before his doctor told him he could. Don't make this mistake!

The Later Period

After the first few weeks, you can no longer just take it easy. In fact, it's crucial that you become active. Now is the time to rebuild your muscles and, in particular, to strengthen the trunk extensor muscles (see Figure 8-1). You will need to have special types of therapy to strengthen the spine. You will also need to do back exercises, not only to recover from this surgery but also to prevent further degeneration of your low back and to avoid future surgeries.

Your doctor should have a postsurgical treatment plan for you. Make sure you understand the therapies you need and the exercises you should do. Then be diligent about following this plan, so that you can recover as fully and as quickly as possible.

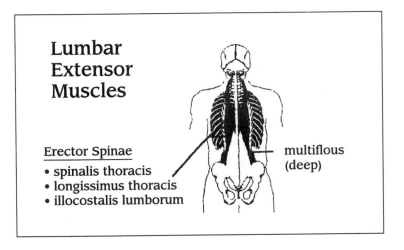

Lumbar Extensor Muscles

Erector Spinae
- spinalis thoracis
- longissimus thoracis
- illocostalis lumborum

multiflous (deep)

Figure 8-1

Proper body mechanics are absolutely essential, not just when you perform your exercises but when you do any movements at all. If your surgeon doesn't have time to instruct you, ask for a prescription to a spine institute or physical therapy center or ask to be referred to an exercise physiologist. You need to understand how to move during everyday activities. Ask the doctor or physiologist to show you how to bend, sit, walk, lift things, get in and out of a car, and so on. Moving correctly is essential to avoiding future injury.

Your exercise program should work to enhance your general fitness, along with the fitness of your back. Some kind of aerobic workout, even if it's just brisk walking, will improve your circulation and your overall fitness level. Although you may be concentrating on strengthening your back, you don't want to ignore the rest of your musculoskeletal system.

Lastly, you need follow-up care. Even if your neurosurgeon doesn't feel that he or she needs to see you regularly, you certainly should be seen by your family doctor or a physician who is interested in spine care. This practitioner will make sure that you are continuing to do well, are still working to strengthen your spine, and are successfully avoiding the deconditioned spine state.

9

Sex and Your Back

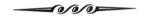

If you suffer from chronic low back pain, the act of sexual intercourse may sometimes cause a flare-up. To cope with this problem, you don't have to take a vow of celibacy. In fact, it's important to note that orgasm can cause your body to release endorphins, natural painkilling chemicals that can ease your overall discomfort and relax your body.

This chapter provides some helpful hints for back pain sufferers who want to remain sexually active. We hope these suggestions will enable you to resume sex with your significant other.

We also recommend that you discuss the issue with your physician. The problem is that this is one of the most difficult topics of conversation for patients—and for some physicians. Patients may very much want to know how they can have an active, healthy sex life when their movements are routinely hampered by low back pain, but they hesitate to ask. In fact, even without any type of back condition, people tend to feel embarrassed about this subject. But try not to be. It's too important to ignore, and the problem won't go away by itself.

Another issue is good communication between you and your partner. If you are in a loving, nurturing relationship, where communication is open at all times, talking to your partner about this issue may not be a problem. However, relationships are never perfect, and for those who have chronic back pain and all of the emotional and lifestyle issues that tend to accompany it, open communication is rarely the norm.

Why? Because it is difficult, even under the best of circumstances, to explain why you're not in the mood for sex. When you know that sexual activities may aggravate your chronic pain, you may feel reluctant to initiate sex, which in turn makes you feel awkward and worried about hurting your partner's feelings.

How do you tell your partner that the intimate acts you have enjoyed together now cause you pain? How do you explain that there is discomfort in your legs or numbness in your feet every time you have intercourse? How do you say that you cannot reach orgasm because of this severe pain?

Another problem is that men with chronic back pain sometimes have difficulty becoming aroused and may find themselves unable to achieve or maintain an erection. And women with back conditions may have difficulty achieving orgasm because they are distracted by their pain. These are very real and very difficult issues.

Why Love Can Hurt

Why does sexual activity increase your pain? If you can think of sex as a form of athletic endeavor, you may find this easier to understand. Consider other physical activities that you are avoiding because of your back pain. Perhaps you don't do housework or yard work, or you've cut back on how often you do them. You may also avoid lifting, even if it's to pick up your two-year-old. You may try to avoid bending, even if it means giving up something you love to do, such as working in your garden. Perhaps you plan your trips to the post office or supermarket for slow times when you won't have to stand for a long period.

Sex is also a physical activity, so even fairly sedentary sex can cause discomfort. The repetitive forward- and backward-bending motions of sex often aggravate back pain, and any type of side-to-side twisting may do the same. (Fortunately, some positions are much less painful than others, and we will describe them later in this chapter.)

Keep in mind that sexual intercourse is a physical act, but sex has important psychological components as well—the anticipation, the sensuality, the emotions. You can have sensual feelings toward another person even if you have ongoing back pain. And you can act on these feelings if you take into account both your own needs and your partner's needs and if you communicate honestly with your partner.

Communication Is Key

Because any activity can aggravate chronic low back pain, it is best if you talk to your partner about which positions and which activities are best for you. If you're unsure, perhaps your partner will help you experiment to find out.

Remember that your partner wants you to experience pleasure, not discomfort, and is likely to feel upset if you don't enjoy yourself during lovemaking. So be sure to tell him or her ahead of time that you have pain with some positions. Don't wait until you're in the throes of passion, when such a discussion is likely to dampen the energy and enthusiasm of the moment. And don't keep the problem to yourself. If you avoid sex altogether because you fear how certain positions will make you feel, you are shortchanging yourself and your partner.

When you have this discussion, you may find that your partner is relieved to learn that it is certain positions you want to avoid rather than him or her. Miscommunication, or noncommunication, may have led your partner to believe that you no longer cared. This talk will probably make you realize that your partner simply wants you to feel good and isn't exclusively concerned with his or her own sexual pleasure.

Physical Modifications

You can adjust your positions and motions during sex in many ways to keep the act from exacerbating your back pain. Try those we recommend. You may find that experimenting a little leads you and your partner to additional experimentation and discoveries that not only prevent your back from hurting but actually enhance your pleasure.

Change Positions Frequently

Don't rely on having intercourse in one way only. The missionary position (face-to-face, with the male on top) is rarely the most comfortable position for a man with low back pain. Changing positions during intercourse can take the pressure off a tender muscle or muscle group. Avoid extremes of bending forward or backward from the waist or middle of the back; this can take the pressure off the nerves and even off the joints.

We recommend lying on your side (see Figures 9-1 and 9-2) as well as lying on your back with support under your knees. You may have already discovered that lying on your back with one or two pillows under your knees is a comfortable way to sleep and one of the few ways to reduce back pain during the night.

Bend or Flex with Your Hips

You can take some pressure off the low back and the pelvic girdle by bending or flexing from the hips (not the waist). Cautiously rock your pelvis, swinging it slightly forward, and see whether this provides some relief.

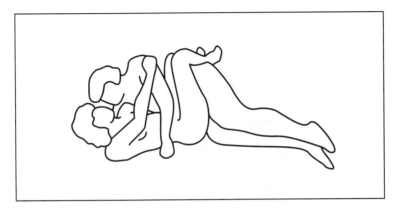

Figure 9-1

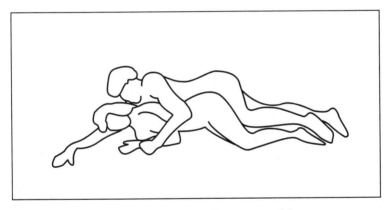

Figure 9-2 Positions in which you lie on your side are easy on the back.

Certain positions make this type of motion easier. The person with the back problem can lie on his or her back while the other person straddles him or her (see Figure 9-3), or the man can kneel in front of the woman while she puts her legs around him (see Figure 9-4).

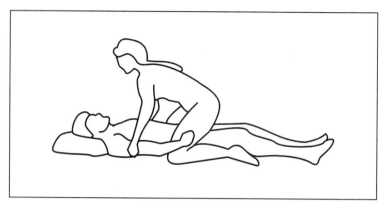

Figure 9-3

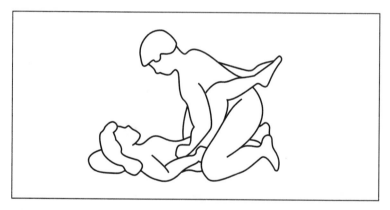

Figure 9-4 Flexing the hips takes pressure off the back.

When Is Sex Possible?

A question that often troubles back pain sufferers more than the how of sex is the when. Specifically, can you have intercourse with your partner when you are having back spasms?

Can you engage in intercourse if you have just recovered from a painful flare-up?

As in any other athletic activity, taking it "slow and easy" is the rule. When you have severe pain, it is certainly not an appropriate time to be having intercourse. Of course, it is also not an appropriate time to play basketball, racquetball, tennis, hockey, or soccer. Balance common sense with sexual needs.

If a flare-up has subsided and you would like to proceed with sexual relations, we suggest that you take this very slowly. Regardless of your performance in the past, marathon sessions are generally not appropriate the first couple of times you try sex after a period of intense back pain.

Test the waters, instead. A brief lovemaking session, in a safe, supportive, nurturing situation, is the best option. It has to be okay for you to say that you can't continue if your pain begins to be aggravated by the activity. We cannot

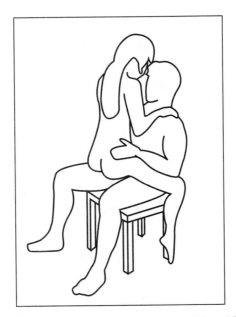

Figure 9-5 Creative sexual expression is possible with a bad back.

stress enough the role that communication plays in sexual intercourse.

Difficulty with Arousal

The knowledge that sex may bring on pain can make it difficult for a man to achieve erection as well as penetration. If he and his partner discuss the matter and accept that penetration is not the mandatory goal of sexual activity, he will feel less pressured, and this alone may ease the problem enough to actually result in intercourse.

But other factors can affect a man's ability to become aroused. For example, he may be on medications that interfere with erection. In addition, past "failures" can lead to the expectation of future inability. It's important for a man to discuss the issue openly with his physician and, when necessary, to consult a urologist.

Women with back problems may also be inhibited by their fear of pain. Furthermore, medications can suppress the desire for sex, and if a woman is internally dry and fearful about how her back is going to feel, intercourse can actually cause pain in the vagina as well as in the back. A woman with this problem should discuss it with a caring and competent gynecologist as well as with her partner. A simple solution, such as using a sexual lubricant or jelly, can sometimes resolve the problem.

Sex Without Intercourse

When intercourse is likely to cause severe pain, willing couples can engage in other sexual activities, such as mutual masturbation, oral sex, or even just touching each other's bodies. At these times, you may wish to concentrate on satisfying your partner, you may want to agree that each of you will concentrate on his or her own pleasure, or you may want to find activities that don't involve penetration but are enjoyable for both of you.

The key, once again, is good communication. When you fear that your back is going to hurt, tell your partner, and together you can discover ways to enjoy each other without causing pain.

10

Sports and Your Back

Before your back trouble began, you may have enjoyed a wide variety of sports, such as golf, tennis, and bowling. Don't think you must forsake these sports because of your back. You may need to modify your movements, develop better skills, and take days off when your back pain worsens, but you don't need to give up playing. Follow our guidelines, and these pleasures can once again be part of your life.

Golf

For some people, golf is the ultimate experience, the pinnacle of achievement, and the essence of life. These individuals live for more than sex, work, and financial rewards: They live to golf! If this sounds like you, what happens if your back pain flares up and it (a) prevents you from golfing, or (b) God forbid, ruins your golf game? This is a question we hear so frequently that we sometimes refer to ourselves as the "golf doctors."

First of all, to understand golf and the back, you need to understand the mechanism of golfing. This sport can put tremendous pressure and strain on the spinal column. Considering the torque, flexion, and extension of the swing, the maneuvers performed by golfers are some of the very worst motions for a healthy spine, let alone a spine that is already in pain.

And that is under the best of situations, when the maneuvers are performed with great skill. A less-than-perfect golfer is truly punishing his or her back. Few of our patients are perfect golfers; they admit that they don't keep their heads down and that they don't have an expert rotation, much less the perfect swing. We often ask our patients to demonstrate their swings, and we see that they not only twist, but they move their necks and backs forward and backward as they follow through.

This is not good. These motions can inflame the joints (facet syndrome) as well as strain the large and small muscles of the low back.

So, what do we tell these patients? And what is our advice for you, if you, too, are an imperfect golfer yet one with a passion for the sport? We certainly don't want you to give up an activity you love. But we do feel that you can't continue to golf with serious flaws in your maneuvers. You must learn to golf in a healthy fashion.

Take Lessons

As in any other athletic endeavor, it is important to get proper instruction. If you have never had golf instruction, we recommend that you see a good professional at least to review your swing and make sure you have the correct body mechanics. Specifically, the pro should make sure that you aren't bending excessively or whipping your torso, and he or she should observe how severely you rotate your trunk during the swing.

We highly recommend taking some lessons, if you have the time and the money for them. Don't assume that because

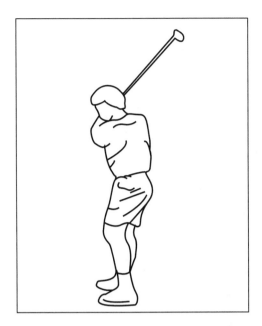

Figure 10-1 The golfing stance must be correct to maintain a healthy back.

you've been golfing for years, you don't need lessons. You may have been making the same mistakes repeatedly over all those years, and you may find that your game improves significantly after just one or two sessions with a good instructor. After all, if you learn the correct mechanics, you'll not only protect your back from aggravation, but you'll also become a better golfer—which is the goal and dream of most people who love golf.

Warm Up

Few people realize the importance of warming up before playing golf. Many of our patients don't perceive golf as an athletic endeavor; they think of it as a social event. But, as any serious golfer will attest, it is a sport. Before starting to

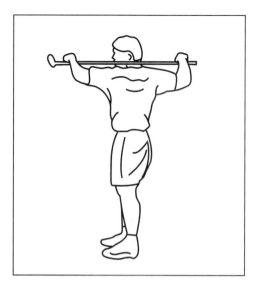

Figure 10-2 A good warm-up is essential.

play, you must warm up your muscles by increasing blood circulation.

A proper warm-up begins with five to ten minutes of an aerobic activity. You can march in place, ride a stationary bicycle, walk briskly, or do anything else that gradually raises your heart rate and warms your body. (If someone else will bring your clubs and the course is nearby, try riding your bike there.)

Follow your warm-up with some stretching exercises to increase your flexibility. We recommend doing those described in chapter 5. In addition, thoroughly stretch your torso—you want to rotate, flex, and extend your spine. Do a simple extension stretch by placing your palms, at hip height, against a wall, and stepping backward until your body is at a ninety-degree angle (bent from the hips, not the waist). You can use a golf club across your shoulders to help rotate the upper torso (see Figure 10-2). When your warm-up includes both aerobic and flexibility exercises, you are most likely to have a safe and enjoyable game.

Jogging

Most people have been told that walking is a good activity to help them get started on an exercise regimen. Better still, they believe, would be jogging. At first glance, this may seem to be a relatively low-risk sport. But you must consider the physics involved in walking and jogging.

As you may recall from chapter 5, your body carries its own weight multiplied by the force of gravity. So each and every step you take transmits a great deal of pressure up and down the spinal column.

If the spine's bones and intervertebral discs, which function as shock absorbers, are working well, there is usually no problem. A healthy individual can walk briskly or jog with little risk of injury, at least to the spinal column. However, if the bony joints have some type of dysfunction (such as arthritis or facet syndrome), or if the discs themselves are experiencing problems (perhaps protrusion, herniation, or aging and loss of fluid), even simple activities such as walking can become painful.

If you have this kind of condition, don't think that you should avoid walking or even curtail how much you walk. And don't decide that you will never be able to jog either. Rather, use common sense, as you would for any other sport. First, a good general warm-up is mandatory. If you're planning to take a brisk walk, warm up with a slow stroll for five minutes, then gradually quicken your pace over another five minutes. Now you can pause to do some stretching and other exercises that move your joints through their habitual range of motion, helping you to feel loose. Finally, you can begin your brisk walk and, if you feel ready and are moderately fit, increase your pace until you reach the speed of a jog.

Wearing good athletic shoes is also very important to preventing injury. Get properly fitted with comfortable, sturdy shoes designed for walking or running, and replace worn-out shoes promptly.

During the first few weeks of your exercise program, allow yourself to walk with a slow yet steady pace. Over time, you can build up to a vigorous exercise level. Remember the adage that we must crawl before we can walk, and walk before we can run. If you have not been athletic in recent years, you should not attempt to jog or even to walk fast on your first outing. Stamina and endurance will increase over a period of weeks, adding to your enjoyment of this activity.

Bicycling

When you're looking for a way to increase your fitness, it's hard to imagine a more safe and harmless sport than bicycling. And yet, if you suffer from back pain, even this simple activity can increase your discomfort, aggravate your syndrome, and possibly even lead to additional degeneration of your muscles, ligaments, and joints. But don't relinquish your interest in bicycling.

Consider the equipment and its effect on your back. If you purchase the best equipment for your body and are careful not to tax your back with lengthier rides than it can endure, you can enjoy bicycling regularly and use it to enhance your physical fitness.

We recommend that you avoid the racing style of bike, which forces you to remain bent far forward. The extreme flexion to reach the handlebars can lead to irritated joints, protruding discs, and serious strain on the low back region. Combine this aggravation with the shock sensations transmitted through the bicycle to your spine when you go over rough roads, and you see that riding a racing bike can have a significantly negative physical impact.

Mountain bikes seem to work much better for people with low back pain. This style of bike has wide, knobby tires, which absorb shock better, and its frame allows the rider to maintain a more upright posture.

Of course, maintaining any posture for a long period of time is unhealthy for the spine and will certainly aggravate the small muscles of the back, particularly if they are already weak. So start out with short rides, and lengthen them gradually to see how much your back can take.

In addition, we need not go into detail regarding the dangers of falling off a bike and all the possible injuries. Anyone who already has an injured back certainly should approach this sport with some degree of caution, particularly if that person is a novice. Wear the proper equipment, and don't ride on roads where motorists may be unable to see you. Stay off rocky or potholed roads, too.

If you're new to biking but interested in pursuing it as a mode of exercise and recreation, we have some suggestions:

1. Have yourself evaluated at a good bicycle shop where knowledgeable people can assess your body frame and cycling experience and help you choose an appropriate bicycle. Physical factors, such as the lengths of your legs and torso, make a big difference in how comfortable a particular bike feels to you.

2. Always use protective gear. Make sure you have a good helmet.

3. Keep in mind that bicycling, while an excellent aerobic activity, does not condition or strengthen the back; in fact, it does very little for the entire upper body. As a result, a general fitness program, including stretching and strengthening work, should supplement your bicycling regimen.

4. Approach your new sport with realistic expectations. During the first weeks, use easy gears and don't push yourself. As you gradually work up to longer and harder rides, you'll find that bicycling can be extremely fun and challenging.

Bowling

Like bicycling, bowling appears to be a fairly low-risk activity. We must point out, however, that lifting and manipulating bowling balls that weigh twelve, fourteen, or sixteen pounds can actually cause a great deal of pain, particularly if your back is already in poor condition.

As we recommended for golf and bicycling, professional assessment of your body mechanics is a good idea. Corrections of your bowling style can lead to an enormous reduction in your low back pain. For example, if the ball you choose is the wrong size for your body, you can actually have a problem both in starting your backswing and in your ultimate delivery. Your spine may rotate too far, and, if one knee is flexed

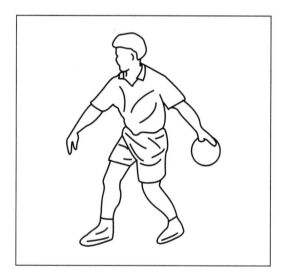

Figure 10-3 Correct form is important in any athletic activity. People who overdo bowling or who use poor form can often feel the pain in their hips, knees, and, especially, low backs. So be cautious, and pay attention to how you feel. As in other activities, "slow and steady" is the motto for every bowler, not just the novice.

and the other bent, there is a great deal of stress on the spine. Together, these forces on the lower back are tremendous and can lead to much inflammation and irritation. But if a pro points out the problem and suggests that you use a lighter or heavier ball, you may discover that your back isn't bothered by bowling the way it once was.

Even if bowling is a social event for you, remember that it is also a serious athletic activity, requiring the same attention to your body as jogging or bicycling. You must do an appropriate warm-up, with flexibility and range-of-motion exercises, and a slow increase in activity. If you have never bowled or haven't bowled in a long time, play for only short periods at first. Even if you used to bowl regularly, you must not return to the sport by immediately playing as many games as you used to play, or you will inflict a great deal of discomfort on yourself.

Dancing

Neither of us is an avid dancer (although one of us has been asked repeatedly by his spouse to take up ballroom dancing), so it's a good idea to consult a dance instructor about the best ways for a person with low back pain to avoid aggravating his or her condition. Nevertheless, we do have a few comments for those who enjoy this activity.

Because the man usually takes the lead, the stress on his low back tends to be greater than the stress on his partner's. Of course, in modern dance this is not always the case. Dance styles have changed over the years, but one thing has remained the same: As the body continuously moves and gyrates, it ultimately goes through, at one time or another, motions that take the joints beyond a natural, comfortable range.

To prevent such movements from bothering or reinjuring your back, we recommend doing a good warm-up, stretching, and starting out with a slow-paced dance. You can then begin to increase the intensity. Be cautious about trying tricky maneuvers, especially if they involve strongly arching the back. As with other diversions, take some lessons if you plan to go dancing frequently.

Football

If you currently have back pain, or your back has ever been injured or chronically painful, we can make only one recommendation: Don't play this sport! Enough said.

Swimming and Water Therapy

We both recommend swimming, essentially without hesitation, to our patients with back pain. Our only strong warning is that those with neck pain, as well as back pain, should avoid hyperextending the spine. This means don't overarch your back.

If you favor breaststroke or freestyle, it is important to avoid a swaybacked posture. We often recommend that our patients wear masks and snorkels to help them keep their heads down and their spines straight. Take this precaution, and you'll find that swimming gives you an excellent workout without exacerbating your back pain. In addition, swimming is a superb cardiovascular exercise. Over time, it will improve your general fitness level and, if you are overweight, help you lose the excess fat and pounds.

Even more than swimming, we recommend low impact water aerobics or other pool exercise. One of the best forms of water therapy is water walking. To do this, you briskly walk back and forth in waist-high water at the shallow end of a swimming pool. The water's buoyancy lifts you up, taking the pressure off your spine, yet you get a good workout because the faster you walk and the deeper the water is, the more resistance you generate. This theory of progressive resistance is what revolutionized the fitness industry in the late 1970s.

(Arthur Jones applied this idea in developing Nautilus weight-lifting equipment and, later, MedX therapeutic equipment.) As your strength builds through waist-high water walking, you can progress to chest-high water walking.

If you find that you like water walking as a mode of exercise, we recommend doing it for twenty to thirty minutes at a time anywhere from four times a week to as frequently as twice a day, seven days a week. You can water walk this often because the exercise is very easy on your joints and entails little risk of injury. These advantages make it a great way for people with chronic back pain to develop their physical fitness.

Tennis

Racket sports such as tennis, squash, and racquetball, as well as handball, were once considered low-risk activities for people with back problems. In reality, any activity that involves the

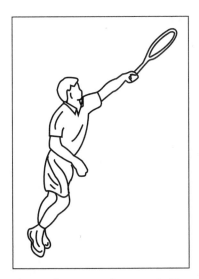

Figure 10-4 You can continue to enjoy tennis if you take care of your back.

movements of these sports—frequent starts and stops, bending and lunging to the side, and extreme extending and flexing of the spine—can certainly aggravate back pain syndromes.

In particular, the extension of the spine with the tennis serve (see Figure 10-4), as well as the follow-through and the accompanying rotation, can put a great deal of pressure on the spine. The whipping motions often seen with topspin forehands, or the two-handed backhand, can inflict too much torque on the spine, producing pain.

For these reasons, you should probably give up your dream of becoming the next Monica Seles or Andre Agassi. But a friendly game of tennis is an enjoyable social activity that your back can tolerate if you follow the basic rules for any athletic endeavor: First, always warm up and do stretching and range-of-motion exercises before you start playing. Second, have an expert evaluate your form and body mechanics.

Your local tennis professional should be able to assess your technique and provide some pointers on how to minimize the risk of exacerbating your back pain syndrome. The advice you'll get is well worth the cost of a few tennis lessons, especially when you consider the high cost of long-term medical care for a back aggravated by playing tennis with improper body mechanics and faulty form.

11

Traveling and Your Back

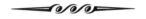

L et's suppose you've followed our recommendations on doctors, exercise, medication, sex, and sports, and your chronic pain is generally under control. But now it's time to go to Grandma's house, and she lives far away. How well does your back travel?

People with back pain need to take special precautions when they travel. Even on a routine trip, you have a higher risk of new injuries to your back as well as aggravation of your chronic pain. After all, you may have to carry luggage, sit for a long time in a seat with poor low back support, or sleep in an uncomfortable bed. When you have a troubled back, the way to travel painlessly is to do some thinking and planning before you leave home. If you consider the possible problems you may encounter and prepare ways to cope with them, you can make it much more likely that you will have a safe, pleasant trip. In this chapter, we offer some suggestions to help you to prepare.

Bring Your Medical Records

We recommend that our patients always travel with their medical records. While this may seem excessive, imagine going to a walk-in clinic in some unfamiliar city, knowing you need a narcotic, muscle relaxant, or prescription pain reliever, but hearing the doctor say, "Oh, it's just a back sprain. Take some ibuprofen, and you'll be fine."

If you have suffered from back pain for years, you know when your pain is serious and requires aggressive intervention. If you travel with records from your neurologist or spine pain specialist, the doctor at the walk-in clinic or hospital emergency room can look at the last treatment that successfully ended a bout of severe pain and take appropriate action.

At the very least, your medical records will prove to the doctor that you are not seeking narcotic thrills, that you are not looking for a quick fix, and that you have had your condition thoroughly assessed and evaluated by a medical specialist.

Pack Intelligently

Consider the best way to pack for the trip you're taking. This may seem trivial, but thoughtful decisions on the little issues can make a huge difference in how you feel during your journey. If you are planning a long weekend away, for instance, you will realize that taking two small suitcases instead of one large overstuffed suitcase can keep you from wrenching your back or having to walk with your torso bent to one side.

In addition, you may want to purchase luggage that is easy to transport. It's often helpful to have suitcases on wheels so you can roll them or a collapsible luggage cart, which you can check with your suitcases. Lifting a twenty- or thirty-pound suitcase can be the worst thing for an individual with back strain, leading to muscle spasm and possibly a protruding or even ruptured disc.

Use the Available Assistance

Pay the skycap at the airport or the bellhop at the hotel. Don't be obstinate or stingy about this. It is amazing how many people will lug their heavy suitcases out of car trunks, having to use all sorts of improper body mechanics to do so, when a skycap or bellhop is a few steps away and even asks, "May I help you?"

Remember, this is their job. Skycaps and bellhops know how to lift and carry luggage without injuring themselves. Take advantage of that!

Change Your Position Frequently

Even people who should know better will often sit through a three-hour plane trip without once getting up to walk in the aisle, stretch, and change positions. When you have to stay in one place for a long time, keep reminding yourself to switch to a different position.

Airplane seats are designed for maximum seating capacity, not for ergonomic comfort. We therefore recommend that you get up after just twenty to thirty minutes, walk up and down the aisle, stretch, bend, and gently twist. If the flight is going to be a long one, take a special orthopedic backrest, which can maintain proper spinal alignment.

If you do use some kind of back support, whether a rolled-up towel or an orthopedic backrest, it is important that your spine is not kept in the same position—even a healthy one—for too long. After sitting for thirty or forty minutes with the backrest in place, get up and walk around. Or, at the very least, take the back support out, so your back can return to its habitual position.

If you are driving to your destination, don't drive for four or five hours straight just so you can get there fast. You may arrive early but also feeling miserable. Stop to use the bathroom and walk around at least every two hours, if not more often.

This little technique will make a big difference in the long run, and it plays an even larger role if you have to remain seated for several days of travel. Where we live in southwest Florida, we see this on a seasonal basis, as travelers from the Midwest come to spend the winter here. They will often drive for two or three days straight, rarely taking the time to get out of the car and move around. After a three-day trip, they may have back pain for two to three months. Then, just when their back pain is essentially resolved, it is time for them to travel back up north. Sadly, they will often repeat the cycle all over again.

Exercise While You're Away

An ounce of prevention is worth a pound of cure. On no matter is this more true than in dealing with spine pain disorders. Doing your exercises to maintain the strength of your back muscles, even while on the road, can be extremely important, particularly in preventing flare-ups.

Don't decide that because you're on vacation, you're not going to exercise. You will not end up having a good time if your back begins to ache. In fact, from what our patients tell us, people with back trouble enjoy their vacations more when they do their daily stretches, take along their swimsuits, and actually do water therapy (see chapter 10) two or three times a week. They feel better in general and do not have to deal with back discomfort.

Please refer to chapter 5 for simple exercises that can greatly reduce or even prevent back pain.

Ask for Boards and Extra Pillows

Dealing with a strange bed—this is a problem you may face frequently, especially if you have to travel for work. How do you keep your back in shape when you must sleep on a soft or lumpy or very hard mattress? If you arrive at a hotel to discover the mattress is too soft, call the front desk and ask to have a board brought to your room and placed under the mattress. Most reputable hotels can fulfill this request.

Better yet, when you are making reservations in advance, specifically request a firm mattress. You might want to explain that you are under a physician's care for back pain and that a firm mattress is very important to prevent aggravation of your condition. Hotel managers, if they have any business sense, will usually try to honor such a simple request.

In addition, when you have a low back problem, certain sleeping positions are better than others. Even if the mattress is poorly designed or badly worn, sleeping on your back with two pillows under your knees and one pillow between them will often provide comfort. You may also find it comfortable to lie on your side with your knees drawn up and a pillow between them.

Give Yourself Time

Our patients tell us that they are constantly rushing on their business trips or vacations and that this stress seems to aggravate their back pain. While this frenzy may be affecting them in a number of ways, one thing we know for sure is that stress seems to intensify back pain.

We therefore recommend that you do whatever you can to limit your physical and emotional stress during travel. Allow yourself plenty of time for everything. Leave for the airport earlier than you normally would. Don't schedule very brief stopovers that will mean you worry about making your airline connection and have to run to do so. Call for taxicabs at least half an hour before you need them, rather than five minutes after you have to be somewhere. And when you're on vacation, remember that you're on vacation: Don't schedule all your free time so that you spend your entire holiday rushing from one "fun" activity to another.

A Man Who Should Know Better

While preparing for a trip, a man we know well has often been admonished by his wife, "Be careful. Don't hurt your back." This person makes a real effort to pack appropriately, taking smaller suitcases, though more suitcases. But occasionally, when traveling with his family, he has to overpack, and on rare occasions, he must take a steamer trunk. The couple has three small children, so you can imagine how much stuff fills this steamer trunk and how heavy it becomes.

Invariably, with the stress and excitement of travel, this fellow will try to lift and haul the steamer trunk himself, using improper body mechanics, and almost inevitably he'll end up with a back sprain or strain. Of course, he never seeks assistance with the luggage and will never allow a sky-cap to help out.

The last word always comes from this individual's spouse, who states, "I told you so." That individual, we must admit, is one of the authors of this book. So, if nothing else hits home in this chapter, remember this one piece of advice: "Listen to your spouse." You'll feel better, and you'll avoid the "I told you so."

Our recommendations are not foolproof and you may have to adjust them to your own situation. But if you use them as a general guide, they can help you navigate your spine pain disorder through many journeys, with both the routine activities and the inactivity that are always part of travel.

12

Women and Back Pain:
Special Considerations

——⟋⟍⟋⟍⟋——

D espite the advances of past decades in equal opportunity
for women, there will always be basic and significant
physiological differences between men and women. Some of
these differences mean that certain kinds of back problems
experienced by women are directly attributable to being
female.

Only women menstruate, and only women can become
pregnant and give birth. Women continue to be the primary
caregivers for children, which is a factor that affects the back.
(They have to carry infants and toddlers, bend to pick up toys,
stoop to zip jackets and tie shoes, and so forth.)

In addition, male and female bodies differ significantly in
terms of fat density, fat distribution, and susceptibility to
changes in bone density, as well as in terms of the changes
that occur with age. In this chapter, we explore some of the
physical changes that women experience, and how some of
them may relate to increased back discomfort.

The Menstrual Cycle

Let's start with the basic changes that first clearly separate women from men. They happen during puberty, when girls begin to menstruate. Hormonal changes generally occur in a cycle lasting twenty-eight or twenty-nine days.

The simple hormone surge before and during menstruation brings such changes to the body as fluid retention, sloughing of the uterine lining (which leads to menstrual cramping and bleeding), and the complex neurochemical changes in the brain that help to regulate this cycle. As it turns out, these changes can have an adverse effect on the low back region.

An interesting study published a number of years ago indicated that women who had endometriosis (growth of the uterine lining in places outside the uterus) also suffered significant low back discomfort during menstruation, stemming from the direct release of the endometrial wall into the abdominal cavity. This problem may lead to scarring and abdominal cramping as well as low back pain from muscle spasms and ligament changes.

Many women experience fluid retention during their menstrual cycles, and this alone can add the extra few pounds that alter the body's center of gravity and consequently increase the stress on the low back and spinal erector muscles. This extra weight can actually trigger muscle spasms and pain in the low back. Many women have found that taking diuretics (pills that help the body release urine) during this phase of their cycle not only alleviates the fluid retention but also reduces their low back discomfort.

The cyclical changes in brain chemicals are a symptom that many people associate with premenstrual syndrome (PMS). Some experts speculate that these chemicals can actually lower the pain threshold so that any existing low back discomfort that seems tolerable during the rest of the month becomes unbearable just before menstruation. Painful states can, of course, lead to irritability or mood changes, which are other difficulties associated with the menstrual cycle.

Pregnancy

The subject of how pregnancy relates to low back pain has been studied extensively. We provide a summary here.

Some studies have investigated which women are at risk for low back pain during pregnancy and which ones actually experience low back pain during pregnancy. One study actually suggested that it would be a good idea for women to look at pregnancy as a twelve-month process, with the first three months being a period of preparation. During this first quarter, they would learn about parenting, but they would also learn about how to improve the condition of their low backs, how to enhance their overall fitness through exercise, and how to create a general state of wellness to help their bodies endure the nine months of gestation. We believe preparing for pregnancy is a wise course of action, and we advise women who plan to have children to consult their doctors before getting pregnant. Find out how to exercise and get your body ready for the back strain that pregnancy can bring. Of course, you can't perfectly time your pregnancy to occur immediately after your period of preparation. But even if the preparation precedes conception by a year, the time you spent enhancing your general health is still likely to be beneficial.

Age

Certain studies of women and pregnancy indicate that younger women are at greater risk for back pain. While the age that separates "older" from "younger" varies from study to study, the general consensus is that the latter category applies to women under thirty. Keep in mind, however, that statistics deal with groups, so individuals' symptoms vary greatly. If you are twenty-six and intend to become pregnant within a year or so, you are not doomed to back pain, especially if you exercise and take sensible precautions.

Kidney Infections

Some researchers have looked at the incidence of pain in the sacroiliac joint that is also associated with kidney infections, under the assumption that pregnancy makes women susceptible to kidney infections. These infections may lead to severe joint pain and inflammation in the low back. This serious problem suggests the importance of careful diagnostic testing, possibly using magnetic imaging of the low back and sacroiliac joint to screen for infections or inflammatory joint problems, and to help determine whether antibiotic therapy is necessary. Physicians must be careful in their selection of antibiotics for pregnant women and may need to consult with a woman's obstetrician.

Changes in the Body

Another interesting study looked at the workload of pregnant women to see whether there was a correlation with muscle and joint complaints during pregnancy. This study focused on the fact that pregnancy actually caused changes in a woman's work activities and work characteristics. With the physical changes that pregnancy brings, the researchers hypothesized, there would be corresponding changes in body position and activities, and possibly an association with workload.

The study revealed that certain facts of pregnancy, particularly the weight gain, change the body mechanics and consequently change the normal load-bearing capacity of the musculoskeletal system. The problem is that the load-bearing capacity is reduced during pregnancy at the same time that stress—the weight that must be carried—increases. In fact, one of the changes to the musculoskeletal system is caused by the body's production of relaxin, a sex hormone that naturally relaxes ligaments and joints (in preparation for childbirth).

This study highlighted the fact that the many changes of pregnancy can lead to low back pain: Not only can changes in both posture and body mechanics give rise to this pain, but also changes in body composition and weight can do so.

Numerous other studies have explored this stress on the spinal erector muscles that occurs during pregnancy. Of course, we know from countless studies that being obese or overweight is a risk factor for low back pain. And, as discussed here, we also know that childbearing, with the forward posture of the abdomen, is a risk factor for low back pain. Taking both of these factors into consideration, a woman and her doctor should carefully monitor her weight gain during pregnancy to minimize, as much as possible, the trauma to the back. Many obstetricians are now recommending a weight gain of about twenty-eight pounds over the entire pregnancy. Gone are the days when doctors felt that more weight gain meant a healthier baby.

Physical Fitness

One study, published in the April 1994 issue of *Spine*, outlined the positive effects of a fitness program that would reduce sick leave during pregnancy and lessen back pain. Researchers found that good physical fitness during the pregnancy and postpartum period actually reduces the risk of low back pain in future pregnancies. This study also noted the need for a careful diagnosis when back pain occurs during pregnancy. For example, among the women studied, it was important for the doctor to differentiate between low back pain and posterior pelvic pain. If a woman had pelvic pain, the study found, she could significantly reduce her discomfort by wearing a supportive garment under her waist.

Researchers in virtually every medical specialty have studied the effects of pregnancy on the low back. One common feature of the results is that a state of general fitness reduces the risk of low back pain, particularly after the first pregnancy. But an exercise program also seems to reduce the severity and frequency of low back pain during a first pregnancy. Various studies have suggested that physical fitness and regular exercise make labor and delivery much easier, although this has not been clearly demonstrated. Some experts even speculate that a general fitness program could reduce or eliminate "back labor," severe back pain that occurs with labor contractions.

Osteoporosis

One fascinating study, published in the October 1993 issue of *Clinical Endocrinology,* studied osteoporosis (loss of bone density and calcium) during pregnancy. The findings suggested that the loss of bone density during pregnancy is much more common than has previously been suspected, although the reasons for this weren't clear. One factor in this loss is probably the hormonal changes that occur during gestation. Because the bones become more fragile with osteoporosis, the rate of fractures increases. In the study, the women with this problem did have an increased rate of spinal fractures. An associated issue is whether there may be a genetic predisposition toward osteoporosis during pregnancy. Follow-up studies are certainly necessary to elucidate the meaning of this study.

Back Pain During and After Childbirth

Many studies have explored back pain during labor and in the months after childbirth. The studies on postpartum back trouble have looked not only at the frequency, intensity, location, and nature of the back pain, but also at whether women who receive epidural injections and anesthesia during labor are more at risk for future back pain.

In one study, published in the May 1993 issue of the *British Medical Journal,* almost 30 percent of the respondents reported having a backache that lasted more than six months after they gave birth. Of these individuals with long-term back pain, 15 percent had no preexisting back problem. In addition, this study indicated that the women who received epidural injections for pain relief were more likely to experience back pain after childbirth, though it tended to be different in quality—more postural and much less severe—from the intractable back pain that lasted many months in other women.

After reviewing the studies carefully, we can conclude that epidural pain relief does not seem to contribute significantly to serious long-term back pain, although it may cause certain women to experience positional back pain for a short period after giving birth.

Another review revealed a possible correlation between the severity of a woman's menstrual pain and the severity of her labor pain. Women who have severe menstrual cramping appear to experience more intense front and back labor pain than do women whose cramps are less debilitating. In addition, women with serious menstrual cramping also report a higher degree of continuous back pain during labor.

According to one interesting study, published in *Pain Magazine,* episodic low back pain that is not associated with menstrual cramping is also not associated with increased labor pains. Researchers had formerly believed that women who had experienced menstrual cramping as well as periodic low back pain before their pregnancies were at greatest risk for complaints of severe labor pains.

Other research has revealed that the position of the mother during labor is correlated with the severity of her low back pain. During labor, safely changing the woman from lying on her side or back to a vertical position (sitting or standing) seemed to greatly reduce the intensity and persistence of her low back pain. This change in position seemed to be most helpful during the first stage of labor, which is notoriously the longest phase.

Macromastia

When large-breasted women develop a number of symptoms, such as headache, neck pain, shoulder pain, pain beneath the line of the bra straps, and back pain, the condition is called macromastia. Women with large breasts have a center of gravity that is high and forward in their bodies, which commonly leads to increased strain and torque on the low back muscles, particularly the spinal erector muscles, whose strength is important in reducing back pain syndrome. Also, in this posture, the pelvis tends to tilt backward, which can increase back discomfort, especially at the sacroiliac joint.

One possible solution for women with macromastia is an operation to reduce the size of their breasts. Among a number of studies on this topic, one that appeared in the January 1995 issue of *Plastic and Reconstructive Surgery* showed that 97 percent of large-breasted women who were to have breast-reduction surgery reported having three of the pain complaints listed in the previous paragraph. Following breast reduction, 100 percent experienced a significant reduction in their symptoms, while 25 percent no longer had any pain whatsoever. However, the degree of improvement in back pain did not clearly reflect the volume of breast tissue that had been removed, for reasons that are as yet unclear.

If you have large breasts and believe they may be contributing to your back pain, discuss the problem with your physician. Ask him or her about all your options. While surgery to reduce breast size may seem to be a relatively simple solution to a complex problem, we want to stress that this is rarely the sole cause of a back problem. Furthermore, we recognize the social, emotional, psychological, and physical ramifications of this surgical procedure, and we urge you to consider the many alternatives. The cosmetic surgery literature makes this sound like a quick and easy solution, so we want to remind you that it is still surgery, with all of surgery's risks and consequences.

Osteoporosis

As the baby boomers (born between 1946 and 1964) age, osteoporosis will increasingly become the scourge of modern women—unless they take care of themselves. In this condition, which affects women much more often than men and is related to an inadequate calcium supply, the bones lose mass and density, becoming porous and weak. Brittle bones often lead to back pain, and, of course, they break more easily than strong bones, so that someone with osteoporosis may break a bone in a minor fall that would leave someone else unharmed. We have seen patients who had severe back pain from tiny fractures in the spine caused by compression as well as from joint changes caused by the bones' loss of density, all of which can be traced to osteoporosis.

Humans are the only creatures on earth that experience osteoporosis. We attribute this ailment to improper body mechanics, musculoskeletal stress, hormonal changes, environmental changes, and upright body posture. The sedentary lifestyle of most human beings is certainly a risk factor for the progression of osteoporosis.

As we mentioned earlier, certain women seem to have a higher risk for calcium loss during pregnancy than others do, though the reasons are unclear. There may be a genetic tendency toward developing osteoporosis. However, as women age, they are all at risk for loss of bone density and for developing osteoporosis, which is a silent but potentially disabling illness. Endocrinologists (physicians who specialize in hormonal and chemical changes) have performed many studies on osteoporosis. They generally agree on the following facts:

- When hormone production declines because of menopause (especially early menopause) or surgical removal of the ovaries, osteoporosis can begin or accelerate. (Many physicians recommend estrogen replacement therapy to protect menopausal women from osteoporosis.)

- The tendency toward osteoporosis may be inherited. So if your mother or grandmother had it, consider yourself at risk.

- Exercise appears to be extremely effective in reducing or reversing the effects of osteoporosis.

Along with the good news about exercise, new medications to treat osteoporosis are being developed and tested all the time. A recent study, which appeared in the November 30, 1995, issue of the *New England Journal of Medicine,* described the effect of a new medication on bone mineral density and the incidence of fractures in postmenopausal females suffering from osteoporosis. Daily treatment with this substance, Alendronate, actually increased the bone mass in the subjects' spines and hips, and throughout their bodies. It also reduced the risk of spine fractures, the risk of vertebral deformities, and the risk of height loss. While this is certainly a very exciting study, more information needs to be obtained on the risks and benefits of this medication versus those of other, more traditional medications, in their various forms.

In addition to back pain, many individuals with osteoporosis will actually have less tolerance for exercise because it tends to bring on pain. The subsequent decrease in activity often leads to chronic disuse atrophy. In this classic cycle of deconditioning, your back hurts, whether due to illness or injury, so you tend to avoid activity. The lack of exercise leads to additional wasting and weakening of the muscle tissues, and this increases the pain. The intensified pain, in turn, causes you to become even less active. Again, your body becomes even weaker and more susceptible to injury. You can see the downward spiral.

Osteoporosis plays a very significant role in chronic disuse atrophy and should be treated aggressively. It is no longer appropriate for a doctor to say, "Well, I guess you're getting old. It's to be expected." With the new medications, calcium replacement therapies, and the knowledge of exercise's effects on aging and bone density, there are good treatments available that can help people with osteoporosis to become active again. Of course, if you don't yet have osteoporosis, planning ahead to avoid the condition is a better idea than hoping to receive effective treatment after it develops.

What You Wear Can Hurt You

Most of us don't think of women's clothing and accessories as potentially harmful, but some of the items that women regularly wear can greatly contribute to back pain. If you walk in spike-heeled shoes every day or lug around a heavy purse or gym bag everywhere you go, you're hobbling your natural posture, throwing off your gait, and overworking certain muscles. Obviously, none of these things is going to make your back feel good.

High Heels

Long considered a problem waiting to happen by physical therapists, orthopedic surgeons, and neurologists, the wearing of high-heeled shoes can significantly aggravate back pain and even cause it to develop. Spike and stiletto heels are particular culprits in this problem, but all high-heeled shoes throw off the body's normal alignment, shift the pelvis, and increase the stress on the legs. Walking in high heels affects gait, balance, and coordination, making their use a definite risk factor for back pain complaints.

We recommend that you wear comfortable, well-cushioned, and well-soled walking shoes, especially if you have to stand or walk for prolonged periods or if your regular activities involve lifting or carrying. While shoe selection may seem trivial, it can make a real difference in how your back feels and in preventing a worsening of your condition. If you must wear shoes with heels, choose among those that are under two inches, and don't stand for long periods.

The Loaded Purse

As our staff and many patients can attest, Dr. Kandel has been known to weigh women's purses. Even though individuals understand intellectually that they should not carry five to ten pounds around on their shoulders every day, these purses have weighed in at as much as twelve pounds, and the patients carry them across their shoulders or even against their necks. Then they call and complain, "My back is going out, and my neck is hurting."

Remember, you need to consider not just the weight of this object that you're carrying, but rather its weight times the distance from the ground times the force of gravity. This explains why the torque on your shoulder and neck is significant. Accompanying this stress is a secondary discomfort in the low back region.

All of these factors—shifting of the body mechanics, imbalance of stress on the joints, and extra weight—work to produce or aggravate low back pain. In addition, "heavy purse syndrome" can also trigger general muscle inflammation up and down the spine.

Occupational Factors

Even with the changing composition of the workforce, women continue to be the primary caregivers for the majority of children in this country, and this, too, is a factor in women's back pain syndromes. Many studies have been performed on the effects of the bending, twisting, and lifting that are inevitable actions for those whose occupation is child care. Other occupations in which women make up the majority of professionals, such as nursing, also tend to involve these repeated movements.

Fortunately, times are changing, with men assuming more of the everyday work of parenting and taking up occupations that have been traditionally performed by women. Yet the times change slowly. And, as we discussed earlier in the chapter, women will always be more susceptible to certain types of low back pain because of their physiological makeup.

Epilogue

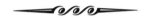

We've talked about why backs hurt, the types of doctors who treat backs, medications, non-pharmacologic treatments, and important exercises. We've also discussed sexual problems related to back pain and how to resolve them, sports you can enjoy despite your condition (if you follow our suggestions), and ways to keep your back happy when you travel.

The message behind all of this is that you *can* get relief from back pain. It is not something that you are doomed to suffer for the rest of your life. You will, however, have to make an effort to help yourself. We and our fellow physicians cannot rid the world of back pain, but we can educate you on how you can improve your condition and work with your doctor.

We hope that you—and your back—are better off for having read this book.

Frequently Asked Questions

QUESTION: *I am forty to forty-five pounds over my ideal body weight. Tests have shown that I have a herniated disc in my low back, and I'm losing muscle strength and greatly troubled by severe pain. My doctor says I'm too overweight for surgery and that my risk of a good surgical outcome is poor. He urges me to lose weight and says we can then discuss the possibility of surgery. What should I do?*

ANSWER: A study at the Medical College of Wisconsin in Milwaukee addressed this issue. Researchers compared people who were overweight (more than 20 percent above their ideal body weight) to people who were at their ideal weight. The obese group comprised twenty-eight men and twenty-seven women. The results of how the patients felt after back surgery looked like this:

	Obese Group	*Normal Weight Group*
Excellent	38%	42%
Good	38%	39%
Fair	18%	12%
Poor	7%	7%

As you can see, the outcome for the obese group was about the same as that of the normal group. The duration of surgery and blood loss appeared to be slightly greater for the obese group, while the length of hospital stay and complication rates were essentially identical.

While physicians agree that obesity is undesirable in patients with low back pain, it should not be an obstacle to surgery for those who have a compelling need.

QUESTION: *I suffered a back sprain approximately two years ago. I was fairly active in the past, but I find myself no longer able to jog, lift weights, and engage in other conditioning activities. As a consequence of this, I have gained about forty pounds. How dangerous is this?*

ANSWER: It could be fatal. A recent study in the *New England Journal of Medicine* has identified body weight as a very significant risk factor for mortality. In middle-aged women, excessive weight was found to be a contributing factor in death from all causes. Women with normal body weight were not found to have high death rates from the same ailments. It's also worthy of note that the lowest death rates among middle-aged women were among those who weighed 15 percent less than the national average.

These findings should be enough to motivate you to take charge of your back problem, follow the advice in this book, and resume exercising with a suitable program.

QUESTION: *Does a stressful lifestyle contribute to the development of low back pain?*

ANSWER: A recent Finnish study, reported to the International Society for the Study of the Lumbar Spine, suggests that stress does play a role in low back pain. The findings were based on an enormous number of participants (8,000), with 100 percent follow-up over a period of ten years.

More than 1,100 of these individuals applied for a disability pension at some time during the period of observation. Researchers found that heart attack was the most common reason among men who applied, while for women it was unspecified chronic low back pain. People who scored high on the mental stress scale were 164 percent more likely to apply for government aid than those with a normal stress score. It's interesting that among those who claimed a disability based on a specific diagnosis, such as lumbar stenosis or herniated disc, this back problem did not appear to be related to the mental stress quotients. Hence we may surmise that while severe stress is unlikely to rupture a disc in your back, it may help to stir up pain when there is no structural abnormality.

QUESTION: *Can excessive alcohol consumption or cigarette smoking be related to low back pain?*

ANSWER: Beyond the well-known and thoroughly documented roles of alcohol and tobacco in various diseases, there does appear to be a relationship between low back pain and alcohol abuse or smoking. Both cigarette smoking and heavy alcohol use are definite risk factors for osteoporosis, a very common and disabling ailment that can cause low back pain.

A recent study of 9,704 independently living, Caucasian, 65-year-old women found that those who smoked were generally weaker, had poorer balance, and performed less well on tests of physical functions than did those who did not smoke. The same study, however, suggested that moderate drinkers had generally better physical function than nondrinkers. Moderate drinking was defined as fewer than fourteen drinks per week.

Cigarette smoking is also a significant risk factor for degeneration of the intervertebral discs. This habit also detracts from general physical fitness, which is important in people with chronic back pain.

QUESTION: *I have a large hump in my upper spine, just at the base of the neck. My mother and aunts had similar deformities. What causes this?*

ANSWER: The deformity you have described, often called a "dowager's hump," is the single most common abnormality of osteoporosis affecting the spine. It is thought to be caused by small fractures in the vertebrae of the thoracic spine, as well as by weak extensor muscles (the back muscles on either side of the spine).

An interesting study originating from the Mayo Clinic suggests that increasing the strength of the extensor muscles can actually lessen this deformity. We recommend that you discuss a suitable exercise program with your doctor.

QUESTION: *Although I've never had any bone fractures, my doctor tells me that I have early osteoporosis. (He did some type of scanning procedure that apparently proved this.) He has me on calcium supplements, estrogen therapy, and calcitonin injections. Should I be doing anything else?*

ANSWER: Absolutely! Aerobic exercise, such as brisk walking and bicycling, are good for keeping your muscles and cardiovascular system in good condition, as well as maintaining posture.

Possibly of more importance, however, is weight-bearing exercise, as revealed by findings published in the *Journal of the American Medical Association.* This study looked at the effect of high-intensity strength training (resistance training) on osteoporosis. Forty postmenopausal women, aged fifty to seventy, participated in the study, which involved resistance training twice a week on five different exercise stations. This was a controlled study, with twenty individuals doing the exercise and nineteen not doing the exercise. Bone density scans were performed before and after the twelve-month period of the study. Bone mineral density (a measure of bones' health) was significantly improved in the exercising group.

While it might seem unusual for older people to be using Nautilus machines and the other weight training equipment you see at gyms and health clubs, this study clearly demonstrates the value of this type of exercise therapy in the treatment of a potentially crippling disorder.

QUESTION: *I am a man, twenty-seven years old, and have had back pain for about six months. I was injured at work while lifting heavy boxes. My pain is in the lower part of my back, just to the right of the middle. I have not experienced any leg pain, numbness, or weakness. I have been to a neurosurgeon who says that I have a bulging disc, that nothing can be done, and that I should learn to live with this pain. Is he right?*

ANSWER: People suffering from low back pain should be aware that essentially any structure in the back may be causing their pain. This includes any of the joints, supporting muscles or ligaments, discs, bones, blood vessels, tendons, and even structures in the abdominal wall and the abdomen itself.

The fact that you have a bulging disc does not necessarily mean that it is the source of your discomfort. An article in the *New England Journal of Medicine* relates the results of MRI scans on ninety-eight people with no pain. Amazingly, only 36 percent of these individuals had normal discs at all the spinal levels studied. Even though the individuals with abnormal discs had no symptoms, 52 percent had a bulge at one level and 28 percent had even more significant abnormalities. Furthermore, 38 percent had abnormalities at more than one disc level.

Thus doctors should be very cautious about relating a patient's symptoms to the abnormalities that are found through a study such as an MRI. No one test can pinpoint the source of a patient's pain. In fact, in patients with nonspecific low back pain, the precise location of the pain is often not discovered.

In most cases, the highest level of accuracy is achieved when the physician obtains a good history of the patient's pain, performs a comprehensive physical examination, and uses the results of any necessary tests. He or she then interprets all of this information together, thus looking at the condition in context. Remember, the best physicians treat the patient, not the test! We suspect that much can be done for your low back pain. We suggest that you find a doctor whose orientation in treating chronic low back pain is based on the judicial use of stretching and strengthening exercises.

QUESTION: *I injured my back approximately six months ago in an automobile accident. I had no head or neck injuries that I could identify and felt no pain from these sources until approximately six to eight weeks after the accident. Since then, I have had severe pain in my neck, as well as headaches. Does this make any sense, or am I crazy?*

ANSWER: It is well known that headaches and neck pain can come in the wake of a low back injury, even when no specific injuries are identified to the higher regions. This is a well-documented phenomenon whose precise cause is unknown. It may be related to the need of the neck muscles to compensate for the prolonged spasm in the back, or it may be related to the increased emotional stress, including depression, that often follows an injury.

Another possible cause of your pain is any medication you were given after your accident. Many of the medications that are used to treat low back injuries can lead to headaches if taken for a prolonged period. These medications have even been reported as the cause of a noninfectious type of meningitis.

QUESTION: *I injured my back in a car accident two years ago. An MRI showed mildly bulging discs but otherwise was unremarkable. Since the injury, I have had severe low back pain that has not improved despite therapy. (In the same accident, I broke my arm, but that pain disappeared in two months.) I did get a lawyer, and when my case was finally settled, I was left with approximately $2,000 after my medical bills were paid.*

Beyond the suffering from my back pain, I have been divorced and have been forced to take a job that pays much less than my previous position. My children think that I belong in a nursing home. I have had to give up golf, water-skiing, and even boating—all activities that gave me great pleasure. Am I nuts or what?

ANSWER: Your question strikes at the heart of a great dispute that rages among physicians, patients, insurance companies, and the lawyers. Many physicians, defense attorneys, and insurance companies feel that individuals who have chronic low back pain despite treatment are suffering from "compensationitis."

Although we acknowledge that some individuals do attempt to exploit the lawsuit-happy climate in this country, we feel that this is a fairly rare occurrence. Certain studies have suggested that the pain in the back or neck that follows an automobile accident is miraculously cured when a settlement is made, but most of these studies have been flawed by severe bias in their investigational methods.

Scientific studies suggest that even after the patient's suit is settled, the pain persists. As in your case, nonspinal injuries, such as fractures, typically heal without lingering pain, while neck and back pain tend to persist.

A study reported in a 1994 issue of *Spine* suggests that people with neck and back pain from motor vehicle accidents continue to improve despite the presence of ongoing litigation. This study was based on thirty-nine patients who completed pain questionnaires at their first and last visits to the doctor. At the time of their accidents, all thirty-nine of these individuals were employed, and it is interesting that, while only twenty-seven were working at the time of their first visits, thirty-eight had resumed working by the time of their final visits. Testing of their physical function demonstrated improvement in thirty-four of the subjects by the end of their treatment, while only four showed a decline in function. Moreover, these patients showed statistically significant improvement not only with regard to pain and function, but also with decreased reliance on medications.

So, the short answer to your question is no. It's not all in your head. Your pain hasn't persisted just because it took a long time to settle your suit. However, you have recently gone through some dramatic changes in your life, and these stresses may be aggravating your condition. Consult your doctor about developing a treatment plan that incorporates both physical and psychological therapies.

QUESTION: *My neurosurgeon tells me that I need back surgery, but he won't perform the procedure unless I quit smoking. Why?*

ANSWER: We don't know exactly what procedure your doctor is contemplating, but we suspect that it may be a lumbar fusion. It has been estimated that a smoker's risk of nonunion (failure of the bones to fuse) is three to four times that of a nonsmoker. Also, cigarette smoking is a major risk factor for degenerative disc disease.

If you believe the surgery will help your back, quit smoking. (In fact, even if you don't want the surgery, quit smoking. The health benefits are innumerable.) If you've tried to quit other times and failed, get your family or friends to help you, or get into a program.

QUESTION: *What are some of the risk factors for low back pain?*

ANSWER: We have addressed many of them in the chapters of this book. However, a list of basic health-related factors associated with the development of low back pain would include the following:

1. Lack of fitness
2. Smoking
3. Weak back or trunk muscles
4. Being overweight

5. Stress
6. Depression
7. Alcohol and drug abuse
8. Emotional and social problems

QUESTION: *I have had low back pain for many years. It comes and goes. Over the last few years, I have seen a neurosurgeon who told me that I don't have a problem he can fix with surgery, an orthopedic surgeon who recommended an exercise program, a family doctor who suggested I take painkillers when my condition flares up, and a chiropractor who told me I should see him on a regular basis. What should I do?*

ANSWER: This is a much more complex question than it might appear to be. Many medical specialists, general practitioners, and nonmedical therapists treat spine disorders and low back pain. Their expertise is concentrated in somewhat different areas, and, of course, skills and knowledge vary from person to person.

We advise you to do the following:

1. Find a practitioner with whom you have a good rapport.

2. Before you start his or her treatment plan, ask three questions: "What is the immediate expected outcome?" "Will it be temporary or lasting? "What long-term results should I expect?"

3. Understand no single therapy works for everyone. If one therapy provides you with moderate relief, maybe combining it with other therapies or modifying the helpful therapy would provide even greater relief. Explore the possibilities with your physician in an open and rational fashion.

An article in the October 1995 issue of the *New England Journal of Medicine* offered a comparison of patients seeing family care physicians, chiropractic physicians, and orthopedic physicians. The three groups of patients had similar outcomes, with the patients seeing chiropractors showing slightly more improvement and/or giving a higher rating to their overall health care.

This goes to show that there are many ways to achieve the same result. We urge you to spend some time and put some effort into finding the method that works best for you.

Glossary

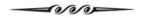

abscess. Collection of pus, infection.

acupuncture. A type of therapy using special needles placed at specific sites on the body in order to release the brain's pain-relieving chemicals.

adhesions. Areas where organs become attached as a result of scar formation.

aneurysm. An abnormal, bubblelike expansion of an arterial wall that is caused by vessel weakness.

anterior. Front side.

arachnoiditis. Scarring and inflammation of the nerve roots in the spinal column, often causing intractable pain. This sometimes occurs because of postsurgical scarring.

atherosclerosis. Narrowing of the arteries with plaque build-up, often associated with high cholesterol levels and a family history of the problem.

atrophy. Loss of muscle mass. This can be related to disuse but is more profound if caused by nerve damage.

bed rest. Limitation of activity, effective only for the first, very acute phase of back pain.

biofeedback. A type of therapy in which a person learns to manage his or her own pain through conscious mental control.

bone plug. Material used in spine fusion; can be obtained from the patient's body or from other sources.

bone scan. A test to determine whether there is hidden inflammation or irritation of bone material.

bone spurs. Calcium overgrowths, often seen on the bony spine, that can irritate the nerve roots.

cartilaginous. Composed of cartilage, which is a tough but pliable material found in the ears and nose as well as on the ends of the bones inside the joints.

CAT scan. Computerized axial tomography scan; a diagnostic test that produces an image of the internal structures of the body, including the bones and organs.

cervical. Pertaining to the neck.

chiropractic. A popular type of therapy that emphasizes manipulating the joints to restore a more full range of motion. Recent studies suggest that this therapy may be very effective in the treatment of soft tissue injuries.

chronic disuse atrophy. Muscle shrinkage due to decreased use, associated with long-term illness or pain.

cryotherapy. A treatment in which ice is applied to relieve pain and reduce inflammation; the cold constricts blood vessels.

deconditioned spine. A spine that is weak from disuse. This can lead to additional deconditioning or injury and is often part of a chronic pain syndrome.

discogram. A fairly painful study that provides information about the low spine's disc material. In this test, a contrast agent (material that can be seen on x-rays) is placed inside a disc prior to taking x-rays.

disc transplant. An experimental surgical procedure that has had some positive results in animal studies and may be a possibility in the future.

diskitis. Infection of an intervertebral disc.

dural sac. Tough membrane surrounding the spinal cord.

electromyography. See EMG.

electrophysiologic test. Electrical test performed by a neurologist in a neurologic laboratory to evaluate the nerve function and muscle function of the spine and legs.

EMG. Electromyography; the muscle study that neurologists perform to determine whether there is muscle inflammation or nerve root inflammation.

epidural. Literally means "surrounding the sac of the spinal cord"; often used to mean epidural injection, a pain-relieving injection into the space around the spinal cord sac.

evoked potential. A sensory type of electrical test used to determine impulse transmission by a particular nerve or in a particular area of skin.

facet block. Injection of medication into a facet joint to produce pain relief. Usually a steroid and an anesthetic are combined.

facet joints. The joints where one bony spine structure interlocks with another bony spine structure; often a source of significant pain in the low back region.

facet syndrome. Inflammation of a facet joint; can lead to severe low back pain.

fibromyalgia. A condition marked by inflammation of the muscles, ligaments, and tendons.

fibromyositis. Inflammation of the main, fleshy part of a muscle as well as the surrounding ligaments and tendons.

This term is frequently interchanged with the term *fibromyalgia.*

fibrosis. Scarring.

flexibility training. Instruction in maneuvers that can increase the function and range of motion of muscles and joints.

herniated disc. Ruptured disc; the gelatinous inner core of an intervertebral disc has broken through the tough outer shell. Can pinch or irritate nerves.

herniated nucleus. Similar to herniated disc.

herniated nucleus pulposus. The technical term for ruptured disc.

inflamed disc. See diskitis.

intervertebral disc. The shock-absorbing material between two vertebral bodies of the spinal column.

intractable pain. Pain that cannot be controlled with standard measures. Some physicians may prescribe narcotics for a brief period to enable a patient to cope with this pain.

iontophoresis. A type of physical therapy involving the application of electric current and locally applied medication. It can relax muscles and reduce pain.

lamina. A part of the bony vertebral body that is sometimes removed during surgery on an intervertebral disc (see laminectomy).

laminectomy. Surgical removal of a lamina, creating more space in this segment of the spinal column, in order to relieve compression of a nerve root.

low back strengthening program. The ultimate treatment for a weakened and inflamed spine, particularly helpful in preventing reinjury.

lumbar. Pertaining to the low back.

lumbar canal stenosis. See lumbar spinal stenosis.

lumbar nerve roots. Nerves in the low back that join up to form the large sciatic nerves, which can refer pain to the legs.

lumbar spinal stenosis. Narrowing of the spinal column of the low back, caused by wear and tear.

lumbosacral spine. The lower section of the spine, including the sacrum.

magnetic resource imaging. See MRI.

massage. A therapy involving manipulation of the muscles by hand. It is useful for soft tissue injuries and myofascial pain, and to increase blood flow to inflamed regions.

medical history. The part of an appointment with a doctor in which he or she asks questions in order to form a detailed account of patient's illness, with special attention to factors that make the problem better or worse.

metastatic. Cancer that has spread within the body from an original source to another area.

MRI. Magnetic resonance imaging; the scan that allows a physician to see the soft tissue structures of the body without invasive techniques.

muscle relaxants. Medications used to reduce spasm.

muscle weakness. Loss of strength in a particular muscle group.

myelography. A diagnostic test in which dye is injected into the spinal canal and x-rays are taken to determine whether there is nerve or disc damage.

myofascial pain. Pain related to the myofascial sheath, often felt as diffuse aching, deep burning, soreness, or a nagging sensation.

myofascial sheath. The covering of the muscle belly. It has a very poor blood supply and can remain inflamed long after the muscle inside it heals.

narcotic. A controlled class of medication used for management of intense pain.

neoplasm. Malignant tumor.

nerve block. Local injection near a nerve to reduce pain along the course of the nerve.

nerve root. Small clump of nerve fibers that exits the spine between two vertebrae; carries impulses from the brain to the muscles and sensory information from the body to the brain.

nerve root injury. Any event that damages the nerve root.

neurologist. Medical doctor who specializes in diseases of the nervous system.

neuropathy. A disease process that affects nerves. It is often painful and can produce numbness and weakness, usually in the legs.

neurosurgeon. Neurologic specialist who performs surgery to treat spine and other nervous system disorders.

noradrenaline. A chemical messenger of the brain.

NSAID. Nonsteroidal Anti-Inflammatory Drug; this class of medicines includes aspirin and ibuprofen as well as prescribed medications and is used primarily for pain relief.

nucleus pulposus. The jellylike substance inside an intervertebral disc.

opioid analgesic. See narcotic.

orthopedic surgeon. Bone doctor, often dealing with the major and minor joints of the body, occasionally involved in spine and back care.

orthotic device. A brace or other supportive item that a patient can wear. Used to assist the musculoskeletal system, often during an acute phase of treatment.

osteoarthritis. Wear-and-tear changes, usually of a degenerative nature, in the bony structures of the spine.

osteomyelitis. Inflammation and infection of the bony structure of the spinal column.

osteoporosis. Loss of minerals, especially calcium, from the bony spine as well as the body's other bones.

Paget's disease. A chronic illness in which the bones weaken and become deformed. This is often associated with nerve pain within the bones.

paraclinical. Refers to testing above and beyond the exam done in the clinic. This could include laboratory tests, diagnostic studies, x-rays, or imaging scans.

paraspinal musculature. The muscles on either side of the bony spine.

pedicle. A section of the bony vertebral body.

percussion tenderness. Acute sensitivity to being tapped. Refers to muscles.

peridural fibrosis. Scarring around the sac that contains the spinal cord and nerve roots; often occurs after low back surgery.

physiatrist. Rehabilitation specialist; often treats people who have had strokes or amputations; occasionally deals with spine disorders and spine rehabilitation.

pinched nerve. A nerve that is entrapped by disc material, bone spurs, narrowing of the spinal column, or another process.

postural training. Activities that help the body assume and maintain proper, healthy positions.

radiculopathy. Inflammation of a nerve root, i.e., the origin of the nerve near the spinal cord. Can be caused by a slipped disc, a bone spur, or another problem.

reflex sympathetic dystrophy. A painful condition usually affecting a limb. Most often caused by nerve injury.

renal toxicity. Potentially leading to irritation or inflammation of the kidneys. This may be a side effect of certain medications.

rheumatologist. Medical specialist who deals with joint disease, inflammatory processes of muscles, and problems with tendons and ligaments; often treats people with rheumatoid arthritis.

ruptured disc. The gelatinous material inside an intervertebral disc has broken through its capsule.

sacroiliac joint. The joint between the pelvis and the tailbone. This may become inflamed and is often a source of pain.

scoliosis. Abnormal curvature of the spine.

serotonin. A chemical messenger of the brain.

spasm. Involuntary contraction of muscle tissue. This is a normal, protective response to injury.

spina bifida occulta. A congenital disorder marked by incomplete fusion of the bony spine. This is usually not associated with neurologic dysfunction, although it may be associated with back pain.

spinal fusion. During surgery, neighboring vertebral bodies are actually joined together to lend stability and reduce nerve pain. The fusion is intended to be permanent.

spinal meningitis. A viral or bacterial infection of the spinal canal. The membranes around the brain and spinal cord become inflamed, and there is usually associated back and head pain as well as fever and prostration.

spinal stenosis. Narrowing of the spinal canal, often associated with irritation of the nerve roots or spinal cord. This can produce numbness and tingling, burning, and occasionally weakness in the legs.

spine center. A place that is dedicated to the treatment of spine disorders, usually offering specialized therapy or treatment plans.

spinous process. The projection from the bony vertebral body. These processes are the bumps along your spine that you can feel through your skin.

spondylolisthesis. Fracture of a part of the bony spine. This can lead to excessive rotation or instability of the spine.

spondylosis. The medical term for wear-and-tear arthritic changes of the spine.

steroid. A medicine used to reduce inflammation; often has negative side effects.

subluxation. Abnormal, painful displacement of the bony portions of a joint, i.e., being "out of joint." The term is used primarily by chiropractors.

TENS. Transcutaneous Electrical Nerve Stimulation; a type of therapy that uses electric stimulation to block pain sensations.

thermography. A study that determines whether there is a temperature difference between one part of the body and another. This can indicate inflammation.

thoracic. Pertaining to the midback.

traction. A type of therapy that employs weights and harnesses to stretch the spine. This can reduce back pain, disc protrusion, and nerve compression by realigning the spinal column.

transverse process. A part of the bony vertebral body; a transverse process sticks out on either side of the spinous process and serves as an attachment site for muscles and ligaments.

tricyclic antidepressants. Medications named for their three-ringed molecular structure; they affect the chemical messengers of the brain to ease pain and depression.

trigger block. A type of therapy in which an area of muscle that is tight with miniature spasm is given an injection to provide relief.

ulcer disease. Often called a peptic ulcer; the linings of the stomach and intestine are inflamed and irritated.

ultrasonography. An ultrasound study that uses radio waves to measure the structure of soft tissues.

ultrasound. A type of therapy that applies high-frequency vibrations to muscles to induce relaxation and reduce inflammation.

Bibliography

Anderson, G. "The epidemiology of spinal disorders." *The Adult Spine: Principles and Practice,* edited by J. Frymoyer. New York: Raven Press, 1990.

Anderson, G. and Svensson, H. "The intensity of work recovery in low back pain." *Spine,* 8:880–84, 1983.

Antonakes, J. "Claims costs of back pain." *Bests Review,* 1981.

Beimborn, D. and Morrissey, M. "A review of the literature related to trunk muscle performance." *Spine,* 13:655–60, 1988.

Biering-Sorensen, F. "A prospective study of low back pain in a general population, I: occurrence, recurrence and etiology." *Scandinavian Journal of Rehabilitative Medicine,* 15:71–79, 1983.

Blair, J. A., M.D. "Preinjury emotional trauma and chronic back pain: an unexpected finding." *Spine,* 19 (10):1144–47, 1994.

Bogduk, N., Ph.D. "A universal model of the lumbar back muscles in the upright position." *Spine,* 17 (8):897–913, 1992.

Borenstein, D.G. and Wiesel, S.W. *Low Back Pain: Medical Diagnosis and Comprehensive Management.* Philadelphia: W.B. Saunders, 1989.

Cady, et al. "Strength and fitness and subsequent back injuries in firefighters." *Journal of Occupational Medicine,* 21:269–72, 1979.

Carpenter, et al. "Effect of 12 and 20 weeks of resistance training on lumbar extension strength." *Physical Therapy,* 71:580–88, 1991.

Carpenter, et al. "Quantitative assessment of isometric lumbar extension net muscular torque." *Medicine and Science in Sports and Exercise,* 23:S65, 1991.

Chaffin, D. "Human strength capability and back pain." *Journal of Occupational Medicine,* 16:248–54, 1974.

Chapman, A. "The mechanical properties of human muscle." *Exercise and Sports Science Reviews,* 13:443–501, 1985.

Cherkin, D., Ph.D. "Physician views about treating low back pain, the results of a national survey." *Spine,* 20 (20):1–10, 1995.

Cowley, Geoffrey. "Melatonin mania." *Newsweek,* pp. 60–65, November 6, 1995.

Cunningham and Kelsey. "Epidemiology of musculoskeletal impairments and associated disability." *American Journal of Public Health,* 74:574–79, 1984.

Delorme, T. "Restoration of muscle power by heavy resistance exercises." *Journal of Bone and Joint Surgery,* 27:646–62, 1945.

DeVries, H. "EMG fatigue curve in postural muscles: a possible etiology for idiopathic low back pain." *American Journal of Physiological Medicine,* 47: 1968.

Deyserling, et al. "Isometric strength testing as a means of controlling medical incidents on strenuous jobs." *Journal of Occupational Medicines,* 22:332–36, 1980.

Dillard, et al. "Motion of the lumbar spine: reliability of two measurement techniques." *Spine,* 16:321–24, 1991.

Duckro, P. N. "Migraine as a sequel to chronic low back pain." *Headache,* 34:279–81, 1994.

Dunn, E. F., et al. "Pregnancy associated osteoporosis." *Clinical Endocrinology,* 39 (4):487–90, October 1993.

Egerman, R. S., et al. "Sacroiliitis associated with pyelonephritis in pregnancy." *Obstetrics and Gynecology,* 85 (5 Part 2):834–35, May 1995.

Egoscue, P. *The Egoscue Method of Health Through Emotion.* New York: HarperCollins Publishers, 1992.

Ernst, E, M.D., Ph.D., Letter to the Editor, "Treatment of acute low back pain." *New England Journal of Medicine,* 1786–87, June 29, 1995.

Esses, S. I. *Textbook of Spinal Disorders.* Philadelphia: J.P. Lippincott, 1995.

Farfan, H. "The biomechanical advantage of lordosis and hip extension for upright activity." *Spine,* 3(4):336–42, 1978.

Farrell, et al. "Second chance: rehabilitating the American worker." *Compensation & Benefits Management,* 1989.

Foster, D and Fulton, M. "Back pain and the exercise prescription." *Clinics in Sports Medicine,* 10:197–209, 1991.

Frymoyer, J., et al. "Epidemiologic studies of low back pain." *Spine,* 5:419–23, 1980.

Frymoyer, J., et al. "Risk factors in low back pain: an epidemiological survey." *Journal of Bone and Joint Surgery,* 65:213–18, 1983.

Gonzalez, F., et al. "Reduction mammoplasty improved symptoms of macromastia." *Plastic and Reconstructive Surgery,* 91 (7):1270–76, June 1993.

Graves, et al. "Effect of training frequency and specificity on isometric lumbar extension strength." *Spine,* 15:504–9, 1990.

Graves, et al. "Effect of training with pelvic stabilization on lumbar extension strength." *International Journal of Sports Medicine,* 11:403, 1990.

Graves, et al. "Quantitative assessment of full range-of-motion isometric lumbar extension strength." *Spine,* 15:289–94, 1990.

Hainline, B. "Low back pain in pregnancy." *Advances in Neurology,* 64:65–76, 1994.

Hart, L., Ph.D. "Physician office visits for low back pain frequency, clinical evaluation, and treatment patterns from the U.S. national survey." *Spine,* 20 (1):11–19, 1995.

Hebert, L., P.T., *Sex and Back Pain,* second edition. Bangor, ME: Impact U.S.A., 1992.

Heckman, J.D., et al. "Musculoskeletal considerations in pregnancy." *Journal of Bone and Joint Surgery,* American volume, 76 (11):1720–30, November 1994.

Herno, O., M.D., et. al. "Surgical results of lumbar spinal stenosis: a comparison of patients with or without previous back surgery." *Spine,* 20 (8):964–69, 1995.

Itoi, E., and Sinaki, M. "Effect of back-strengthening exercise on posture in healthy women 49 to 65 years of age." *Mayo Clinic Proceedings,* 69:1054–59, 1994.

Jackson, C., and Brown, M. "Analysis of current approaches and a practical guide to prescription of exercise." *Clinical Orthopaedics and Related Research,* 179:135–144, 1983.

Jackson, C., and Brown, M. "Is there a role for exercise in the treatment of patients with low back pain?" *Clinical Orthopaedics and Related Research,* 179:39–45, 1983.

Jenner, J. R. and Barry, M. "Low back pain." *British Medical Journal,* vol. 310, no. 6984, 929–32, April 8, 1995.

Jensen, M. C. "Magnetic resonance imaging of the lumbar spine in people without back pain." *New England Journal of Medicine,* 331:69–73, 1994.

Jonsson, B., M.D., et. al. "The straight leg raising test and severity of symptoms in lumbar disc herniation: pre-operative and post-operative evaluation." *Spine,* 20 (1):27–30, 1195.

Kandel, J., and Sudderth, D. B., *Migraine—What Works!* Rocklin, CA: Prima Publishing, 1995.

Katsuura, A., M.D., et al. "Experimental study of intervertebral disc alografting in the dog." *Spine,* 19 (21):2426–32, 1994.

Katz, J., M.D., et al. "Clinical correlates of patients' satisfaction after laminectomy for degenerative lumbar spinal stenosis." *Spine,* 20 (10):1155–60, 1995.

Kelly, G. "Effects of aerobic and normo-tensive adults: a brief meta-analytic review of control clinical trials." *Southern Medical Journal,* 88 (1):42–46, January 1995.

Kere, et al. "Outcomes of care of acute low back pain among patients seen by primary care physicians, chiropractic physicians, and orthopedic surgical specialists." *New England Journal of Medicine,* 333 (14):913–17, October 1995.

Kirkaldy-Willis. *Managing Low Back Pain.* New York: Churchill Livingstone, 1988.

Kulig, et al. "Human strength curves." *Exercise and Sports Science Reviews,* 12:417–66, 1984.

Lewith, G. T. *Acupuncture: Its Place in Western Medical Science.* Wellingborough, England: Thorsons Publishers, 1982.

Liberman, U. A., et al. "Effect of oral alendronate on bone mineral density and incidence of fractures in postmenopausal osteoporosis." *New England Journal of Medicine,* 333 (22):1437–43, November 30, 1995.

Liemohn, et al. "Unresolved controversies in back management: a review." *Journal of Orthopaedic and Sports Physical Therapy,* 9:239–44, 1988.

Macek, C. "Neurological deficits, back pain tied to endometriosis." *Journal of the American Medical Association,* 249 (6):686, February 11, 1993.

Malmivaara, A., M.D., et al. "For treatment of acute low back pain—bed rest, exercise, or ordinary activity." *New England Journal of Medicine,* 332 (6):351–59, February 9, 1995.

Malone, T., ed. *Evaluation of Isokinetic Equipment.* Baltimore: Williams and Wilkins, 1988.

Manniche, et al. "Intensive dynamic back exercises for chronic low back pain: a clinical trial." *Pain,* 47:53–63, 1991.

Manson, J. E., et al. "Body weight and mortality among women." *New England Journal of Medicine,* 333 (11):677–85, 1995.

Marras, et al. "Measurements of loads on the lumbar spine under isometric and isokinetic conditions." *Spine,* 9:176–88, 1984.

Max, M. "Antidepressants as analgesics." *Progress and Pain Research and Management,* vol. 1, pp. 230–43. Seattle: IASP Press, 1994.

Maye, L. and Greenberg, B. "Measurements of the strength of trunk muscles." *Journal of Bone and Joint Surgery,* 4:842–56, 1942.

Mayer, H., M.D. "Spine update: percutaneous lumbar disc surgery." *Spine,* 19 (23):2719–23, 1994.

Mayer, H., M.D., et al. "Quantification of lumbar function, part 2: sagittal plane trunk strength in chronic low back patients." *Spine,* 10:765–72, 1985.

Mayhew, T. and Rothstein, J. "Measurement of muscle performance with instruments." *Measurement in Physical Therapy,* edited by J. Rothstein. New York: Churchill Livingstone, 1995.

Melleby, A. *The Y's Way to a Healthy Back.* Piscataway, N.J.: New Century Publishers, 1982.

Melzack, R., et al. "Labor pain: effect of maternal position on front and back pain." *Journal of Pain and Symptom Management*, 6 (8):476–80, November 1991.

Metropolitan Life Insurance Company, Statistical Bulletin, vol. 76, p. 26, April/June 1995.

Miller, A. P., et al. "Breast reduction for symptomatic macromastia: can objective predictors for operative success be identified?" *Plastic and Reconstructive Surgery*, 95 (1):77–83, January 1995.

Murray, A. and Harrison, E. "Constant velocity dynamometer: an appraisal using mechanical loading." *Medicine and Science in Sports and Exercise*, 18:612–24, 1986.

Murray, D. "Optimal filtering of constant velocity torque data." *Medicine and Science in Sports and Exercise*, 18:603–11, 1986.

Nelson, H. D., et al. "Smoking, alcohol and neuromuscular and physical function of older women." *Journal of the American Medical Association*, 272 (23):1825–31, December 21, 1994.

North American Spine Society's Ad Hoc Committee on Diagnostic and Therapeutic Procedures. "Common diagnostic and therapeutic procedures of the lumbosacral spine." *Spine*, 16:1161–67, 1991.

Ostgaard, H. C., et al. "Influence of some biomechanical factors on low back pain in pregnancy." *Spine*, 18 (1):61–65, January 1993.

Ostgaard, H. C., et al. "Postpartum low back pain." *Spine*, 17 (1):53–55, January 1992.

Ostgaard, H. C., et al. "Prevalence of back pain in pregnancy." *Spine*, 16 (5):549–52, May 1991.

Ostgaard, H. C., et al. "Previous back pain and risk of developing back pain in future pregnancy." *Spine*, 16 (4):432–36, April 1991.

Panjabi, et al. "How does posture affect coupling in the lumbar spine?" *Spine*, 14:1002–11, 1989.

Parkkola, R. and Kormano, M. "Lumbar disc and back muscle degeneration on MRI: correlation to age and body mass." *Journal of Spinal Disorders*, 5:86–92, 1992.

Parnianpour, et al. "The triaxial coupling of torque generation of trunk muscles during isometric exertions and the effect of fatiguing isoinertial movements on the motor output and movement patterns." *Spine*, 13:982–91, 1988.

Paul, J. A., et al. "Workload and musculoskeletal complaints during pregnancy." *Scandinavian Journal of Work, Environment and Health,* 20 (3):153–59, June 1994.

Polatin, P. "The functional restoration approach to chronic low back pain." *Journal of Musculoskeletal Medicine,* 7:17–30, 1990.

Pollock, et al. "Accuracy of counterweighting to account for upper body mass in testing lumbar extension strength." *Medicine and Science in Sports and Exercise,* 23:S66, 1991.

Pollock, et al. "Effect of resistance training on lumbar extension strength." *American Journal of Sports Medicine,* 17:624–29, 1989.

Pollock, M., Ph.D., et al. "Muscle." *Rehabilitation of the Spine,* edited by S. Hochschuler, H. Cotler, and R. Guyer. St. Louis: Science and Practice Mosby Books, 1993.

Pope, M. "A critical evaluation of functional muscle testing." *Clinical Efficacy and Outcomes in the Diagnosis and Treatment of Low Back Pain,* edited by J. Weinstein. New York: Raven Press, 1992.

Pope, et al. *Occupational Low Back Pain.* St. Louis: Mosby Year Book, 1991.

Prentice, C., et al. "Back school programs: the pregnant patient and her partner." *Occupational Medicine,* 7(1):77–85, January-March 1992.

Rayna, J. Jr., M.D., et al. "The effect of lumbar belt on isolated lumbar muscles: strength and dynamic compacity." *Spine,* 20 (1):68–73, 1995.

Reynolds, J., M.D., consultant. *Lumbar Disc Surgery, Treating Low Back Pain and Sciatica.* San Bruno, CA: Krames Communications, education booklet, 1990.

Risch, et al. "Lumbar strengthening in chronic low back pain patients: psychological and physiological benefits." *Spine,* 18:232–38, 1993.

Rungee, J. L. "Low back pain during pregnancy." *Orthopedics,* 16 (12):13–44, December 1993.

Russell, R., et al. "Assessing long-term backache after childbirth." *British Medical Journal,* 306 (6888):1299–1303, May 15, 1993.

Schofferman, J. "Successful treatment of low back pain and neck pain after a motor vehicle accident despite litigation." *Spine,* 19:1007–10, 1994.

Schwarzer, A., M.D., et al. "The sacroiliac joint and chronic low back pain." *Spine,* 20 (1):31–37, 1995.

Smidt, et al. "Assessment of abdominal and back extensor function: a quantitative approach and results for chronic low back patients." *Spine,* 8:211–18, 1983.

Snook, S. "Low back pain in industry." *Symposium on Idiopathic Low Back Pain,* edited by A. White and S. Gordon. St. Louis: Mosby Year Book, 1982.

Spengler, et al. "Back injuries in industry: a retrospective study. 1. Overview and cost analysis." *Spine,* 11:241–45, 1986.

Spine Letter, "Disc transplantation: a likely alternative to fusion." Vol. 2, no. 10, October 1995.

Spine Letter, "Is there sex after surgery?" Vol. 8, no. 10, October 1993.

Spine Letter, "Long-term study of mental stress, low back pain." Vol. 2, no. 9, September 1995.

Spine Letter, "Lumbar spine surgery not contraindicated in obese patients." Vol. 2, no. 1, January 1995.

Spine Letter, "Preventing peridural fibrosis." Vol. 2, no. 8, August 1995.

Tigley, M., M.D., "Laser discectomy: a review." *Spine,* 19 (1):53–56, 1994.

Tite, G., M.D., et al. "Outcome after laminectomy for lumbar spinal stenosis." *Journal of Neurosurgery,* 81:699–706, 1994.

Tollison, C. D., ed. *Handbook of Pain Management,* second edition. Baltimore: Williams and Wilkins, 1994.

Tucci, et al. "Effect of reduced frequency of training and detraining on lumbar extension strength." *Spine,* 17:1497–1501, 1992.

U.S. Department of Health and Human Services. "Acute low back problems in adults." AACPR publication no. 95-0642, December 1994.

Videman, T., et al. "Low back pain in nurses and some loading factors of work." *Spine,* (4):400–404, May-June 1984.

Vo, P., M.D., et al. "The aging spine: clinical instability." *Southern Medical Journal,* 97 (5):S26–35, May 1994.

Wall, P. D. and Melzack, R. *Textbook of Pain,* third edition. London: Churchill Livingstone, 1994.

Wiesel, S. W.; Feffer, H. L.; Borenstein, D. G.; and Rothman, R. H. *Industrial Low Back Pain: A Comprehensive Approach,* second edition. Charlottesville, VA: The Mitchell Company, 1989.

Wilder, D. G., Ph.D., et al. "Are chronic back pain patients at risk from unexpected load on the spine?" *Back Letter,* 10 (8):89, August 1995.

Index

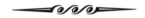

About the Authors

Joseph Kandel, M.D., is the founder and medical director of the Neurology Center of Naples in Naples, Florida, and cofounder of the Gulfcoast Spine Institute. An avid student since his youth, he attended Ohio State University as a Batelle Scholar, obtaining a double major B.S. in zoology and a B.S. in psychology, both with honors. Kandel graduated from Wright State University School of Medicine in Dayton, Ohio, in 1985, where he was president of his freshman medical school class. He completed his residency at the University of California Irvine Medical Center.

Kandel is a popular public speaker and has been published in such prestigious medical journals as *Neurology, Vital Signs,* and *American Zoologist.*

He lives in Naples with his wife and their three children.

David Sudderth, M.D., is the senior partner at the Neurology Center of Naples and is cofounder of the Gulfcoast Spine Institute in Naples, Florida.

He graduated from medical school at the University of Copenhagen in 1984 and completed his residency at the Medical College of Wisconsin and Emory University. Dr. Sudderth accomplished a one-year fellowship in nerve and muscle disorders at Emory University in 1988.

An in-demand lecturer, Sudderth speaks frequently on medical topics. He also produced the popular video *Spinal Tips* and has published in *Neurology* and *Ugeskrift For Laeger.*

An avid computer fan, Dr. Sudderth can often be found perusing the Internet and other computer services, adding to his extensive knowledge of neurological issues and problems.

Also by Drs. Kandel and Sudderth

Spinal Tips: Physician's Home Remedy for Back or Neck Pain
Videotape runs 46 minutes / $19.95 + $3.95 shipping and handling

Chronic back and neck pain sufferers—you don't gain from pain! Get past the pain and enjoy your life again by following the expert, practical, and immediately usable advice found in *Spinal Tips*. The video features simple exercises demonstrated by average people (not athletes or sports specialists) that will help you feel markedly better!

Relief from Hand and Arm Pain: Carpal Tunnel Syndrome and Repetitive Stress Injuries
Videotape runs 16 minutes / $14.95 + $3.95 shipping and handling

Millions of people suffer from hand and wrist problems. If you are among them, this video can help greatly improve your problem or alleviate it all together! Drs. Kandel and Sudderth offer important preventive measures and easy exercises you can integrate into your daily life. Also included are valuable descriptions and demonstrations of tests doctors perform to detect repetitive stress injuries of the hand or wrist, as well as a discussion of surgical options.

NEW! **Migraine News**, a bimonthly newsletter, offers the very latest news, information, and helpful hints for people suffering from migraine headaches, as well as information for their caring family members. Authored six times a year by Joseph Kandel, M.D., and David Sudderth, M.D., this newsletter is must-have reading for male and female migraineurs of all ages.

You'll gain powerful and important medical information in an easy-to-read format—information translated from medical jargon into plain, practical language. *Migraine News* is available now for $18.95 (non-U.S. orders, add $10 payable in U.S. dollars). Order now, and be among the aware and healthy!

Order from:
Pain Management Publishing
8380 Riverwalk Park Blvd., Suite 320
Fort Myers, FL 33907

For credit card orders, call 1-800-844-7880